Discover Your Thinner Self

Discover Your Thinner Self

A Common-Sense Approach for a Slimmer, Healthier You

David Medansky

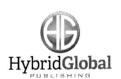

HybridGlobal
PUBLISHING

Published by
Hybrid Global Publishing
301 E 57th Street, 4th fl
New York, NY 10022

Manufactured in the United States of America, or in the United Kingdom when distributed elsewhere.

Medansky, David
Discover Your Thinner Self: A Common-Sense
Approach for a Slimmer, Healthier You
LCCN: 2017958390
ISBN: 978-1-938015-84-7
eBook: 978-1-938015-85-4

Cover design: Leslie Akin/The Brand Boss

Copyediting: Penny Hill

Proofreading: Ayse Yilmaz, Patrick Hodges

Interior design: Medlar Publishing Solutions Pvt Ltd., India

Photo credits: David Medansky, Debbie Medansky

www.BeyondLosingWeight.com

To your weight reduction success for a slimmer, healthier you.

Dedication

For my wife, Debbie,

and

To all the people who failed to lose weight and to those who have lost weight only to gain it all back. I want to thank you for purchasing a copy of this book. I know that by spending your money to make the investment in this, you are putting your trust in me. I fully understand and respect that your time is valuable and that you have many choices for diet and weight-reduction books. I'm honored that you have chosen to read this book. Woody Allen is credited with saying, "Eighty percent of success is showing up." So, thank you for making the effort and showing up.

Rick Frishman usually tells his audience at his *Author 101 University* workshops, "A book can change a person's life." It is my sincere hope that this book might change your life.

Bob, for the record, you were right.

Disclaimer

Before implementing any weight-reduction program, or using any dietary, exercise, or health advice from this book, consult with a qualified health and/or medical practitioner.

All information presented in this book is intended for educational purposes. Any health or diet advice is *not* intended as medical diagnosis or treatment. Statements contained in this book have not been evaluated by the Food and Drug Administration.

The author, publisher, and any other person involved in producing this book disclaim all liability or loss in conjunction with the content provided herein, as well as any and all liability for products or services mentioned or recommended in this book. The information contained herein is subject to personal research and has been recorded as accurately as possible at the time of publication. Due to possible changes and availability of information provided to the public, you should not take any of the content as a source of reference without further research.

If you think you are suffering from any medical condition, you should seek immediate medical attention.

Results may vary: Causes for being overweight or obese vary from person to person. No individual results should be seen as typical.

> **WARNING** – Losing weight using a low calorie or restricted diet can promote crankiness and irritability.

Table of Contents

Introduction . . . . *xv*

Chapter One
A Rejection of Common Sense: Why Being Overweight
or Obese is the New Normal 1

Chapter Two
Weight-Reduction Code of Honor 7

Chapter Three
Weight-Reduction Programs 11

Chapter Four
My Transformational Journey. 25

Chapter Five
Motivation 37

Chapter Six
Commitment to Reducing Weight. 45

Chapter Seven
Eating Environment. 57

Chapter Eight
Stress Makes You Fat 65

Chapter Nine
Weight-Reduction Goals 73

Chapter Ten
Declarations to Reduce Weight 79

Chapter Eleven
Helpful Suggestions for Healthy Weight Reduction 81

Chapter Twelve
High Protein for Weight Reduction. 91

Chapter Thirteen
Weight-Loss Principles 97

Chapter Fourteen
Common Miconceptions 103

Chapter Fifteen
Vitamins and Minerals. 109

Chapter Sixteen
Foods to Avoid. 113

Chapter Seventeen
Summary of Steps to Healthy, Sustainable
Weight Reduction 119

Chapter Eighteen
Success Stories 121

Chapter Nineteen

Final Comments. 127

Chapter Twenty

Beyond Losing Weight. 131

Appendix

A1   Declarations to Reduce Weight. *135*

A2   Sample Weight-Reduction Code of Honor *136*

A3   Recommended Books *138*

A4   Contact Information for Weight Reduction Programs *140*

A5   Example of a Weight-Reduction Diary Sheet *141*

A6   Foods to Avoid to Help Reduce Weight. *143*

A7   Low-Carb/Low Glycemic Load Vegetables *145*

A8   High-Carb/High Glycemic Load Vegetables *147*

A9   Low Glycemic Load Fruits *148*

A10 High Glycemic Index Fruits *149*

Shift Your Mindset to Achieve Better Health *151*

About the Author *157*

Buy More, Save More. *161*

Acknowledgements *163*

Introduction

Do you need or want to lose ten, twenty, thirty, fifty pounds, or more, but you can't get on NBC's smash reality television show, *The Biggest Loser*? For me, I didn't need to lose more than sixty pounds, so I never would have qualified as a contestant. I had to find another way to be a big loser.

Like me, most people who need to lose weight, but not extreme weight, find it difficult to get help. Let's be honest, weight reduction and exercise programs are expensive, time consuming, or require more discipline than most individuals, including myself, have. Generally, individuals who want to shed weight aren't motivated enough or committed enough to do something about it.

I've been where you are. I know what it's like. So, who am I and why should you listen to me? My name is David Medansky, and I succeeded in doing what you're about to attempt. I wasn't always fat. Truth is, for most of my life, I was fit and trim. But, as with many of us, life got in the way. I got lazy and self-indulgent. I stopped exercising regularly and started eating more junk food. Without realizing it, the weight crept up on me.

I was uncomfortable. I was embarrassed and disappointed in myself. I tried and tried but couldn't stop eating or stay on a diet. Instead of eating one scoop of ice cream, I'd eat an entire pint in one sitting. I was disgusted with myself. I couldn't believe my pants size had ballooned up. But I just didn't have the motivation to do something about it.

In July of 2016, I weighed 217 pounds. When my annual physical blood work results came in, my doctor told me to either lose weight or find a new doctor because he didn't want me dying of a heart attack on his shift. With that sword hanging over my head, I made the decision to shed my unwanted and unhealthy pounds. Over the next four months, I lost more than 50 pounds, over 25 percent of my total weight.

I believe it's my duty and obligation to help others lose the weight they need to or want to, so they don't suffer like I used too. As of the date of finishing this book, I weigh 167 pounds. And it feels great. I have more energy. I don't need to nap every afternoon.

I decided to write about my weight-reduction journey and incredible transformation so I could help others achieve their weight-reduction goals. The first piece of advice I'll share with you is this: losing weight is one of the most difficult things you can do. I'll never tell you it will be easy. It's not. But, if I can do it and others have done it, you can do it too!

Nobody undertakes a weight-reduction program to fail. Yet, many do fail because their weight reduction is only a temporary fix. If you're going to discover your thinner self, you'll need to make lifestyle changes.

There are many paths to success. Some people I know have used different dietary/weight-reduction programs with similar results as mine. Others were not so successful. They either cheated or gave up after a few days. W. Edwards Deming stated, "Eighty-five percent of the reasons for failure are deficiencies in the systems and process rather than the employee. The role of management is to change the process rather than badgering individuals to do better." Perhaps people fail to successfully lose weight because they are using the wrong system or method best suited for them. This was so eloquently stated by Evelyn Tribole, MS, RD., and Elyse Resch, MS, FADA, in their book *Intuitive Eating* when they wrote, "In spite of the fact that 90 to 95 percent of all diets fail, you tend to blame yourself, not the diet! Isn't it ironic that with a massive failure rate for dieting we don't blame the process of dieting?"

I wrote this book to be a useful resource for you. You won't find special recipes, exercises to do, or gimmicks. This is not just another *how to* book. It is a *what to do* book. It is written with the intent to inspire you to act now. It explores the mental, emotional, and psychological aspects of losing weight. The continuing theme is motivation and commitment to inspire you to follow through and not quit or give up.

In this book, I share *my* experience. It is not right or wrong, true or false. I am simply sharing *my* experience with you. On the other hand, the information and helpful hints you will learn in this book are based on countless hours of researching the wisdom of some of the greatest mental health professionals, nutritionists, and dieticians around the world. Their revelations have changed tens of thousands of people's viewpoints about how to shed weight and, more importantly, keep it off.

I'm asking you to trust the concepts and ideas set forth in the following pages. Just knowing how to lose weight through the knowledge of what to eat or what exercises to do is not enough. It's not as simple as calories in and calories out. If you properly apply what is presented, the results will speak for themselves. When people deviate from the weight-reduction principles advocated here, do not follow the rules and guidelines specific to each weight-reduction program, and don't change their perspective of food, they fail to lose the unwanted fat. Dropping weight, by melting away fat instead of muscle mass, requires a period of transition. It takes time. Keep the urgency to lose your fat, but be patient.

In the following chapters, I will share with you the tactics that worked for me. If something works for you, then great, keep doing it. Whatever doesn't work for you, toss it out! Does that mean everything I explain about getting rid of weight will work for you?

Of course, not!

All I ask is that you keep an open mind. The weight-reduction strategies, philosophies, and methodologies discussed in this book are not theories. They are proven. I am proof that these techniques work. So are the hundreds of thousands, maybe even millions, of others who have shed weight and kept it off.

Throughout this book, I will refer to weight loss as "weight reduction." The reason being that if you lose something, you tend to want to find it. As you will learn later, this is exactly what happened to many of the contestants on *The Biggest Loser*.

This book is not about nutrition. I'm not a nutritionist. There may be certain foods that worked for me that may not work for you. Or you may have strong feelings about certain foods, being in favor of or against. I'm advocating that everyone has choice. It is up to everyone to make the choices that are best for them. Each person must find their own path to reducing weight and becoming thinner.

I prefer to use the term "weight-reduction program" instead of diet because of the quote, "Athletes eat and train. They don't diet and exercise." Also, people who diet often starve themselves. This is detrimental to the body. I want you to safely get rid of weight in a healthy manner. To me, the word "diet" has a negative connotation because it has the word die in it. I want my message to be positive and uplifting. Diet focuses on seeing food as the enemy, bad eating habits, a temporary fix to the problem, negative aspects of a person's self-image, and a finish line.

Healthy weight-reduction programs should view food as nutrition, fuel for the body. They should teach learning good eating habits, making positive lifestyle changes, making better daily choices, and committing to a life-long journey of maintaining good health. It is not like getting a vaccine where getting one shot covers you for life. It doesn't work that way. Rather, maintaining a healthy weight is a daily, lifetime commitment.

As you read this book, you'll notice that I will repeat things. It is done intentionally so you hear ideas that work several times. Repetition is good for you too, in your efforts. Keep repeating the positive aspects of weight reduction and eating healthy over and over until they become second nature.

It's not easy to reduce weight. The problem is further complicated with all the wrong information and misconceptions out there about how to shed pounds. People think they know what is best, but as Mark Twain stated, "It ain't what you don't know that gets you into trouble; it's what you know for sure that just ain't so." Be wary of people claiming they have the "magic" formula. There is none. If someone tells you they have a secret method to dropping weight, it's a gimmick. There is no amount of money you can pay to get the desired results you want without putting in the time and effort and doing the work.

This book is written to provide you with as much accurate information as possible to make informed decisions. It offers solid, reliable material to help you succeed with your weight-reduction endeavor. Each chapter starts with a bit of advice from me, a saying that expresses the wisdom of the health community, or just a bit of common sense that bears repeating. I hope you find a saying or two to inspire you, to tape on your mirror or fridge.

Making the decision to reduce weight and get slimmer can change your life for the better and improve your overall health. But without following through and persevering during difficult periods, you won't reach your goal. John D. Rockefeller said, "Perseverance… overcomes almost everything." If you act and are tenacious in your efforts, you'll succeed.

If you're ready to stop making excuses and start to shed those unwanted pounds, I wish you success in your journey to reaching your weight goal and discovering your thinner self.

01

A Rejection of Common Sense: Why Being Overweight or Obese is the New Normal

Making the decision to reduce weight can change your life for the better and improve your overall health.

—Common Sense Wisdom

How many people would rather suffer the consequences of poor health, major medical ailments such as cancer or Type II diabetes, or even death rather than give up their bad eating habits to lose weight?

You'd be surprised.

Each year, an estimated 43 million Americans start diets. In 2013, more than 108 million Americans were trying to lose weight or dieting. Americans spend $66.3 billion each year on weight-loss products, purchasing everything from diet pills, to meal plans, to swanky gym memberships. Yet, more than two-thirds of Americans are still either overweight or obese. According to the U.S. Centers for Disease Control and Prevention, 155 million Americans are overweight. Loosely translated, that's more than 71 percent of American adults. Of those who are overweight, almost 40 percent are clinically obese. Being overweight is an American epidemic!

Society and various media have endless ways of making people feel bad about their bodies, and therapists do a robust business helping folks address those feelings, yet America's weight problem persists. Something else is going on.

"It's not your fault." Robin Williams spoke these words playing the role of psychologist Sean Maguire in the movie *Good Will Hunting*. In the scene, Robin Williams repeated to Will Hunting, played by Matt Damon, "It's not your fault," over and over and over until Will breaks down crying and for the first time realizes it's not his fault. So how does this relate to people who are overweight? Simple. It may *not* be your fault.

Researchers are learning that the body will sabotage any effort to lose weight, and worse, to keep it off in the long term. Studies done over the years have found that 80 percent of people who lose weight gain it back. The body will fight like hell to get the fat back. This depressing fact can deter the most motivated dieter to give up. There's the feeling, "Why bother if I'm only going to fail?"

The average weight loss for contestants on *The Biggest Loser* is 127 pounds, or about 64 percent of their body fat. Over time, the average contestant regained 66 percent of the weight they lost. A few gained more than they initially lost.

A study reported in the March 7, 2017, *Journal of the American Medical Association* (JAMA) noted that fewer people are trying to lose weight. Researchers studied data for the period between 1988 and 2014 and concluded: "Socially acceptable body weight is increasing." Why? Because individuals are content with their weight. They are unaware their lifestyles are killing them or that being overweight has severe health-related consequences. Thus, they are less motivated to shed those unhealthy pounds.

Many who are aware of the risks of being overweight or obese are not inclined to do anything about it. It begs the question: why do so many people choose not to act to shed those unhealthy pounds?

Let's face it, it's easier to keep eating the same unhealthy food and avoid exercising. It takes less effort than making a complete lifestyle change. Reducing weight is so hard that many people simply don't want to make any effort whatsoever. But that's not all. According to Dr. Tiffany M. Powell of the University of Texas Southwestern Medical Center, another reason overweight folks see no need to lose weight is because they misperceive their body size. Too many individuals look around and see other overweight and obese people, and therefore they see it as the norm. It's a troubling dichotomy. While people can see they are not supermodels, they think they're healthier than they actually are. I know, that's the image I had of myself.

Doctor Powell suggests that physicians ask patients how they perceive their size and whether they feel they need to lose some weight before talking to them about lifestyle changes. If a person doesn't think they need to lose weight, chances are they won't make any effort to do so. Self-perceptions are changing because overweight and obesity are so common. That's a consequence of America's obesity epidemic: the perception of what is normal has shifted. It's a rejection of common sense.

In this politically correct society, many people believe you shouldn't do or say anything to make overweight people feel uncomfortable. Even physicians walk a fine line. They don't want patients to have an unhealthy body image, but haven't figured out how to make them understand the need to get rid of weight without offending or appearing insensitive. Today's doctors don't want to intervene. The amount of effort required to understand the patient's needs for weight reduction is more than many doctors are willing to put forth. Instead, they're content to write you prescriptions for medication and manage symptoms rather than address your underlying issues. It's much easier for them to prescribe medication than take the time to help a person change their lifestyle.

Further, some of these same physicians are overweight and don't see a need to help their patients. One overweight doctor I met while vacationing with my wife boasted that most of his patients weighed 300 to 400 pounds. And, we wonder why there's an epidemic of people being overweight? Perhaps we should listen to Robert Kiyosaki who said, "Stop taking advice from people more messed up than you."

Intervention is problematic because weight is such a sensitive issue for most people. After all, how many men feel awkward if their wives or girlfriends ask, "Does this make me look fat?" If the husband or boyfriend is truthful, the woman's feelings are hurt. It's easier to not be honest and tell her, "You look great." Unfortunately, the wives and girlfriends probably were also afraid to say anything about the man's expanding waistline.

Thankfully, my doctor didn't care about being politically correct or perceived as being insensitive. He flat out told me, "Lose weight or find a new doctor." More about that wake-up call in Chapter Four.

Sometimes it takes someone else to point out the obvious. My friend John was talking to me and another friend, Lyle, about his fifty-plus high school reunion. John mentioned that he and his children had just finished browsing through his high school yearbook when one of his kids said, "Hey, dad, can I see that again?"

"Sure, why?"

His son opened the yearbook and flipped through it. As the pages cascaded, his son pointed out an interesting observation. "Dad, did you notice that all of your high school classmates were thin? There aren't any fat kids."

"No, not really."

Lyle chimed in, "Now that I think about it, there weren't many, if any, overweight kids in my high school either."

Afterward, I went back home and looked through my high school yearbook. Wow, what a revelation. There were only a handful of heavy-set kids, none of whom I would consider overweight.

Yet today, many children in grades K through 12 are overweight. Think about how that affects self-perception.

Unfortunately, overweight or obese adults incorrectly believe that their bodyweight is just fine. It's a vicious cycle. More individuals are becoming obese, more of them are fine with being overweight, they see others with larger bodies, and they become less motivated to shed the extra pounds. It's the new normal.

Reducing weight and becoming healthy is a choice. For those few who choose to shed unhealthy pounds, it usually means having a better, happier, and longer life. Those who decide not to make the effort put themselves at a higher risk for Type II diabetes, high blood pressure, heart attack, stroke, and certain types of cancer. A 2017 study found that obesity now causes more preventable deaths than smoking.

Ultimately, your success will be a combination of the right program for you, the right motivation, and your own commitment. Take my friend Fred as an example. Fred had exercised most of his life. Because he exercised, he could eat a lot of food and not gain weight. He cut back exercising, but kept eating the same amount of food. Although not obese, he was categorized as being overweight. He never tried to lose weight until his late forties. That's when his doctor informed him his blood-sugar levels were elevated and he was pre-diabetic.

Fred learned that his blood-sugar levels were sensitive to his weight. When his weight dropped by five or more pounds, the numbers improved. When he gained five or more pounds, his numbers undesirably changed. Alarmed by his observations, Fred chose to act. He enrolled in a weight-reduction program and implemented what he learned to drop weight in a healthy manner. Fred told me, "It was tough, but not impossible."

He recorded his fat and calorie intake as well as the food and drinks he consumed. He dropped to just under 200 pounds.

Although technically still overweight, he's a lot healthier than at the 250 where he started.

Unlike a lot of overweight or obese people, Fred was not just interested in shedding his extra weight; he acted.

The fact that you're reading this book is an indication you have some motivation to shed those unhealthy extra pounds to become healthy. It makes sense that if you want to lose weight and keep it off, you should study what people who have reduced weight and kept it off have done. I've compiled the wisdom and best ideas I found in my weight-reduction research to help you get going and keep going on your journey.

Never underestimate what you can do. Your mindset is directly related to your weight-reduction success. Be willing to work for what you want to accomplish. If you're not willing to reduce your weight, no one can help you. If you are determined to shed those extra pounds, no one can stop you. Stop rejecting common sense. Stop being part of the new normal.

> Reducing weight is not about what works for everyone else; it's about what works for *you*. There are many possibilities to accomplish reducing weight and healthier eating. Not "one size fits all." The key to weight reduction needs to be highly individualized rather than a fashionable new diet. The weight-reduction program that works best for your next-door neighbor, best friend, or relative might not be the best for you.

02

Weight-Reduction Code of Honor

If we did all the things we are capable of,
we would astound ourselves.

—Thomas Edison

Thousands of books have been written about diet and exercise for regular, everyday people to lose and maintain their weight. There are numerous weight-reduction programs advertised on television, radio, and on the internet. At the grocery store checkout, you'll see hundreds and hundreds of magazine articles written about weight loss—many of them touted on the front cover. Yet, most ignore an incredibly powerful tool: A Code of Honor.

In his book, *Team Code of Honor—The Secrets of Champions in Business and Life*, Blair Singer states, "Those who are successful have a very clear Code of Honor that is easy to understand and is not negotiable or subject to multiple interpretations. It's a strong set of rules that everyone around them agrees to and part of what makes everyone around them successful as well."

To succeed in any weight-reduction program, you will need to be accountable. Make your family, friends, co-workers, and even your doctor part of your team to support your weight-reduction efforts. Although losing weight is something you must do for yourself, that doesn't mean you must do it alone. Dropping those unwanted extra pounds is difficult to do alone. It helps to have a support team to hold you accountable. No one said getting rid of weight is easy. It's not. If someone tells you it's easy, they are lying.

"I'd do anything to lose fifteen pounds, except eat healthy, give up wine or beer, and start exercising." Does this sound like you? I have talked with many people who say they want to lose weight, but they're just not willing to do anything about it. This is exactly why it is so important for you to have your Code of Honor, your rules, and the accountability to stick to it.

Your Weight-Reduction Code of Honor reflects you and your standards. Your waistline will determine if you are abiding by your code.

Share your code with others. If they are willing to abide by your code, and they agree with it, great. If they disagree with it or aren't willing to help you stick with it, they may be the wrong fit for you. For me, I want to be around people who are going to support my weight-reduction undertaking and weight maintenance. You might consider re-evaluating your relationship with the people who won't support you. Be careful of making exceptions. They tend to become the rule. Remember, your Code of Honor is the set of rules you agreed to.

Every person has their own set of rules. Therefore, it's extremely important to have a code to make sure everyone understands you want to play by the rules defined in it, and to ensure others know they must abide by your rules for you to be successful.

Simply desiring to lose weight is not enough. If you want to maximize the amount of weight you get rid of and keep it off, you need to have well-defined, tight rules. Marines have a strict Code of Honor. They need to be rigid because when bullets start buzzing by a person's head, emotion tends to elevate and intelligence decreases. The code is drilled into Marines over and over to keep them together under pressure. It's a matter of life and death. Otherwise, individuals won't do the right thing to protect the team and each other.

While I'm not saying being in battle is the same as reducing weight, for some reducing weight can be a matter of life and death. For others, it could make the difference between enjoying life or living in misery.

I recommend and suggest you sign and date your Code of Honor. It will help keep you accountable. Keep it in a place where you can refer to it quickly and often.

Honor the code and respect the code of others.

> Execution separates the wishers in life from successful people who act. People who take action care enough about their lives and future to do something instead of hoping it will happen.

SAMPLE WEIGHT-REDUCTION CODE OF HONOR

Below is a sample Weight-Reduction Code of Honor. It is based on my personal Code of Honor. You can choose which rules you want to adopt as yours, or you can create your own.

1. Mission. The mission I have chosen is to lose weight in a healthy manner and to keep it off!
2. Be accountable.
3. Adjust my relationship with food to ensure it is viewed as fuel for my body and not as comfort from my emotions.
4. Record everything in a daily journal.
5. Commit to learning about nutrition and better eating habits.
6. Commit to a lifestyle change.
7. Motivate, encourage, and empower others to lose weight, but only if they have a desire to do so.
8. Never impose my standards on anyone else.
9. Never blame others for my failures. I will take 100 percent responsibility for my own success. No justifications! I'll either have excuses or results.
10. Be willing to get called out if I violate the code. My team must be willing to enforce the code.
11. Never judge or pre-judge others.
12. Do not seek sympathy or acknowledgement. I want to lose weight and keep it off for me. Not anyone else. No one can do it for me. I must be willing to do it myself. Note: It's great if you, the reader, have a purpose or reason (some call it "the why") for wanting to lose weight. But the essential point is that it's your choice.

Agreed to by: *David Medansky*

03

Weight-Reduction Programs

If you're tired of starting over, stop giving up.

—Shia Labeouf

All weight-reduction programs work some of the time, but because each person is different, not every program is suitable for every person. One size does not fit all. Do your own research and decide which is most advantageous for you. Take the time and make the effort to learn about various weight-reduction regimens to determine what will work best for you. Each of us has different situations.

Reducing weight is not about what works for everyone else; it's about what works for you. There are many possibilities to accomplish weight reduction and healthier eating. The key is to understand that weight reduction needs to be individualized rather than following a fashionable new diet. The weight-reduction program that works best for your next-door neighbor, best friend, or relative might not be the best for you.

Successful, long-term weight control should focus on your overall health, not just what you eat or how much exercise you do. A thin person can be just as unhealthy as a heavy-set person. Most people understand that if you stop or curtail exercising yet keep eating the same way, you will gain weight.

Although I refer to it as weight reduction, it should be thought of as fat reduction. Too often, people implement unhealthy tactics to reduce weight. An unintended consequence is loss of muscle mass, water, or both. Not fat. You shouldn't necessarily rely on the scale. Your waistline is a more important indicator.

If you decide to participate in any fat-reduction program, here are some questions to ask before you join. Make sure you're making an informed decision before investing your time, money, and energy. If it's not going to be the right fit for you, you'll just end up frustrated and give up. I don't want you to give up becoming healthier and thinner.

1. Does the program offer group classes or one-on-one counseling that will help you develop healthier eating habits?
2. Is the staff comprised of qualified counselors and experienced health professionals, such as physicians, naturopathic doctors, nutritionists, registered dieticians, nurses, psychologists, and exercise trainers? If so, what are their qualifications? Are they certified?
3. Does the program teach skills and techniques to make permanent changes in eating habits to prevent weight gain?
4. What is the plan to keep the weight off once you've lost it?
5. What does the weight-reduction program consist of?
6. Does the product or program have any risks?
7. How much does the total program cost? Are there recurring fees, food costs, or supplemental products? If the program requires special foods, can you make changes based on likes, dislikes, or food allergies?
8. What are the typical results of participants? How much does an average participant lose and how long have they kept off all or part of the weight?

9. Do you need to follow a specific meal plan or keep food records?
10. If you need to purchase special food, drugs, or supplements, will there be any adverse effects with medication you might be taking?
11. Does the program provide exercise instructions? If not, do they recommend exercise instructors or trainers?
12. Is the program sensitive to your lifestyle and cultural needs?
13. Who oversees the program? What are their qualifications? Does a medical doctor or certified health professional run the program?
14. Can the program provide references or any success stories?
15. Is counseling available on how to deal with stress or slipping back to old habits?
16. Does the program provide ways to deal with holiday eating or lack of motivation?

Reducing weight should be as simple as generating a paint-by-number portrait. To create a beautiful hand-painted portrait, a person is given a simple step-by-step formula for each brush stroke and paint choice. The result is generally breathtaking because scientific method guided every action of the painter. Anyone could do the same and get the same results—all you must do is paint by numbers. Shedding weight is the same. Follow the procedures prescribed, eat the foods recommended, drink pure water, and the weight should come off. But, for some reasons it's not that easy.

Understand that no single weight-reduction program is perfect for every person. That is because we are each unalike, unique in our own way. We have different body chemistries, different metabolisms, and other variants that make it improbable to formulate one perfect healthy weight-reduction method for the general population. Just because one successful person says their weight-reduction program worked for them, it does not mean that it will work for you.

Is there more than one way to lose weight and keep it off? Absolutely! Perusing the diet and nutrition section at a local Barnes & Noble bookstore, I saw hundreds of books on diet and exercise. An Amazon search shows more than 50,000 books on health, diet, weight loss, and fitness. As far as I am concerned, the only good weight-reduction program is the one that is healthy and works for you. Nothing else really matters. But, as I mentioned earlier, it is a lifestyle change, and it is not easy. If you do what is difficult to reduce weight, you will be successful. If you do what is easy to lose weight, it will be tough, if not near impossible, to keep it off.

A friend of mine, Diane, started a weight-reduction program shortly after I had lost more than thirty pounds. After three weeks, she'd only lost a small amount of weight. She complained that she should have lost more. As it turned out, she drank a glass of wine with dinner every night and overate when she met friends for lunch. Alcohol is strictly prohibited when losing weight. Diane was either not committed to losing weight or did a poor job of choosing an effective program and following it.

There is no magical fruit, vegetable, berry, or supplement to reduce weight. Don't bother looking for it. It doesn't exist. If reducing weight was easy, there wouldn't be so many books and articles written on how to do it or so many magazines on weight loss and diet published. We'd all be thinner. There are no short cuts to weight reduction and a healthier lifestyle.

Again, the purpose of this book is to inspire people into acting to lose weight and keep it off. I offer solutions and suggestions to shedding those extra pounds. It is up to each individual person to maintain the discipline necessary to succeed.

If a weight-reduction program seems too good to be true, it probably is. Be wary of weight-reduction programs that make false claims such as, "Lose weight without diet or exercise," "Lose weight with certain foods," "Lose weight while you sleep," or "Losing weight is easy." If someone tells you they have a product that can help you lose weight, think about what's in it for them. Ask them what they gain from it. They are most likely just trying to sell you something. The media and talk shows have a record of putting out information on curtailing weight that has been proven wrong. And they don't care because it's all about ratings. Question everything you hear and read about losing weight. Research what is being publicized as the next great fat burner. Make sure it is backed with studies and proof. More importantly, make certain there are no unintended or detrimental side effects that can cause you to suffer poor health. Just because you lose weight doesn't mean you're doing it in a healthy, nutritious manner.

We are all susceptible to claims of a magic pill, secret formula, or special food to produce extraordinary weight-reduction results. The most sought-after solution is often the newest, fastest fat buster available that doesn't require dieting and exercise. I'm sorry to tell you, it doesn't exist. I know because I looked for the magic pill.

The extract, *Garcinia cambogia*, was publicized as the miracle way to melt away fat but later was proven to have no impact on body weight or burning fat. But I bought into the hype. The ad appeared on my computer touting how easy it is to lose weight and burn fat by just taking this miraculous fruit. My prayers had been answered! Immediately, I went out and purchased a bottle. During the next four weeks, I religiously popped the pills.

After four weeks, I hadn't lost any weight. Not one pound. Another disappointment using a weight-reduction product. Of course, what I hadn't realized yet is that I needed to change my eating habits. But they don't tell you this. They make it appear as if you can continue eating whatever you want. This is not true.

Several case studies done in Mexico, Canada, and Latin America found that the Garcinia supplements were linked to liver failure and other harmful gastrointestinal ailments. A case report published in the Annals of Hepatology in 2016 by the Transplantation Center at the Mayo Clinic also reported dietary and herbal supplements, and specifically *Garcinia cambogia*, are most likely connected to acute liver failure. The report stated, "The false assumption that herbal supplements are 'natural' and therefore safe is a common misconception among consumers." The lesson to be learned is to be extremely careful about what is being offered as a quick weight-reduction product.

Why do you want to reduce weight? Is it for health reasons or to look and feel better? Whatever your personal motive is, have a plan and stick to it. Or in many cases, have a program and stick to it. The number one reason people want to reduce their weight is to improve their health. The World Health Organization noted that being overweight is the fifth leading cause of death around the world. More deaths occur because of people being overweight than from smoking.

Are you willing to put in the time and effort to learn how to change your lifestyle, and your relationship with food? If not, then just keep doing what you're doing. The chance of losing weight and keeping it off is exactly zero. You're either serious and totally committed to losing weight and burning fat or you're just not. There is no in-between. People who have been successful losing fat and keeping it off decided to act and stuck to it. Those who failed, didn't.

Howard Schultz, CEO of Starbucks, said, "Success is not an entitlement. It must be earned." The same applies to weight reduction. Reducing weight and keeping it off is based on merit. It must be achieved. Your efforts will determine your results. The fact remains that you must make a conscious decision for a lifestyle change. Without changing your eating habits, you will regain all the weight you lose and in some cases, even more.

Below are just a few of the many different programs for losing weight. You can decide for yourself which of these programs, or any other, is best for you. If you feel that they may be too expensive, too time-consuming, or you don't want to make the investment in yourself, think how much it costs to treat illness. Some of the major illnesses associated with being overweight or obese include, but are not limited to, Type II diabetes, heart disease, stroke, liver failure, high blood pressure, sleep apnea, osteoarthritis, and some cancers.

Isn't it worth the money if it's possible to avoid diseases simply by reducing your weight and improving your health? I know for me, it was a major influence to finally act and get serious about my weight reduction. Besides, most fast food meals cost more than a prepared healthy meal offered by the programs described below.

The programs summarized here have helped millions of people lose weight. If none of these programs is suitable for you, research the many others that are offered and use the list of sixteen questions on page 12 to find one suited to your needs.

Weight Watchers® provides various products and services to assist in weight reduction and maintenance. With over forty-five years of assisting people in getting rid of unwanted weight, Weight Watchers is one program that has stood the test of time. It was started in 1961 by Jean Nideth, a Brooklyn housewife who decided to host support meetings in her home for people wanting to lose weight. It would not have survived this long without proven results. The core philosophy of Weight Watchers is to help participants lose weight by forming helpful eating habits, exercising regularly, and providing support. The Weight Watchers plan creates a calorie deficit menu, but no food is off limits.

According to Weight Watcher's literature, the framework requires participants to measure and limit the quantity of food consumed, whereas other diet plans dictate a range of acceptable food choices. Individuals can participate in a Weight Watchers program either through in-person meetings or online-only. Many of the individuals who have attained prolonged weight reduction with Weight Watchers indicated that attending meetings was the most prevalent reason for their success. According to several studies, people who participate in group programs and attend meetings lose three times more weight than those who attempt to do it on their own.

Weight Watchers is based on the principle of making changes that can be incorporated into any lifestyle. It is not a quick fix. It works to change the way people perceive food. Weight loss change is not so easily put into practice. But Weight Watchers is the zenith of helping people make long-term dietary change.

A benefit to implementing the Weight Watchers program is that although they have their own line of food, you have the option of choosing groceries outside the Weight Watchers product line.

Juice Plus® is an educational company combining three foundational whole food products which get health snowballing in the right direction for cellular repair, rejuvenation, detoxification, and weight reduction, if needed. When I was on an extremely low-calorie weight-reduction plan, I took the Juice Plus raw food capsules to make certain I got enough nutrition to do it in a healthy manner. For those of you who are unaware, wrapped around the Juice Plus products line is a program called Shred 10. It focuses on the four cores toward long-term health, namely: eating real food, drinking plenty of water, exercising, and managing stress. The four basic elements of the plan are to eliminate "toxic" food and substitute meals with low glycemic shakes or bars, increasing fruit and vegetable intake, supplementing with concentrated fruits, vegetables and berries daily, and avoiding sugar. Unlike old-fashioned vitamin supplements, Juice Plus provides whole-food based nutrition from a wide assortment of nutritious fruits, vegetables, and berries.

The three basic elements of the program are: cutting down on calories by substituting meals with shakes or bars, increasing fruit and vegetable intake, and supplementing with juice-based tablets. The supplements are also sold alone as a bridge for people who do not consume enough fruits and vegetables daily.

I believe there are no coincidences in life as I met Rachel Smartt, a Nutritional Counselor of eighteen years, who shared with me this simple tool to get thirty super foods in my body daily. She is a Naturopathic Doctor and Nutritional Counselor who appreciates the independent peer review and clinical research Juice Plus offers. Juice Plus' Shred 10 is a proven, powerful plan for controlling weight, re-routing negative thinking, preventing disease, and extending life.

Jenny Craig® is a program designed to provide structure and support to help members lose weight and learn how to keep it off. Jenny Craig's program provides nutritionally-balanced menus, which include more than 100 delicious entrees, desserts, and snacks developed by dieticians, nutritionists, and food technologists. One-on-one consultations provide general support and education on portion control and strategies such as Fresh and Free Additions, which helps with satiety. Jenny Craig consultants work with each member individually to identify their strengths, challenges, and personal goals to create unique weekly meal and activity plans that fit individual needs. Consultants also help members implement behavioral strategies to support their success.

Jenny Craig's comprehensive approach to weight reduction is available to members either in person in centers or by phone with Jenny Craig Anywhere. Hard science backs the program as demonstrated by a 2010 independent two-year clinical trial published in the Journal of the American Medical Association showing that participants on the Jenny Craig program lost three times more weight than dieting on their own. Jenny Craig, based in Carlsbad, California, is one of the world's largest weight reduction and weight management companies, with approximately 600 company-owned and franchised centers in the United States, Canada, Australia, New Zealand, and Puerto Rico.

Ideal Protein® is a weight-reduction method with a beginning, a middle, and an end. It is a medically designed protocol containing two key components: weight reduction and a healthier lifestyle education to assist the person with maintaining their results after losing the desired weight. It was originally developed by Dr. Tran Tien Chanh, who focused his career on nutrition with an emphasis on the treatment of obesity and obesity-related issues. Ideal Protein describes itself as follows:

• Structured weight reduction while supporting muscle mass
• An understanding of how food affects and is utilized by the body, including what causes fat storage
• Weekly, one-on-one coaching, lifestyle education, and guidance
• Personalized approach to setting weight-reduction goals based on the individual's health profile
• Improvements in blood pressure and blood sugar and cholesterol levels

Nutrisystem® is a commercial provider of weight-reduction products and services. I'm certain you've seen Marie Osmond promoting Nutrisystem on television advertisements and infomercials. This is a meal-replacement program. The company sells its products and programs on the internet and through a call center. Nutrisystem programs are also sold on QVC®, in Costco® stores, Kroger Grocery®, and Walmart® stores. Nutrisystem uses portion-controlled foods and structured meal plans. Behavioral support is not available in face-to-face interaction. They do, however, offer free access to trained counselors via telephone, online chat, and email.

Contact with counselors is only initiated by customers and is not regularly scheduled or required as part of the program.

HCG® is a physician-supervised program developed by Dr. A.T.W. Simeons, M.D. HCG is Human Chorionic Gonadotropin, a hormone produced during pregnancy to help a baby grow. Be careful! Use only a physician-prescribed and administered HCG drops or shots. Synthetic HCG causes extreme hair loss. Almost none of the HCG supplements sold in health food stores or pharmacies contain actual HCG. The HCG plan has two parts. Both are equally important. In the first part, a person takes HCG. Anecdotal evidence suggest that it helps reduce hunger and helps the body burn fat not muscle. The second part is a low-calorie diet with very restricted and limited food choices. Many people refer to it as the "500 calories per day diet." In fact, it's not 500 calories per day, and a person does not count calories. Rather, it is a low-calorie diet. The HCG plan is done in rounds. Each round consists of the following:

1. Two days of fat loading with HCG,
2. Twenty-one or thirty-eight days of low-calorie, restricted food with HCG,
3. Two days of low-calorie, restricted food, but NO HCG,
4. Three to six weeks of maintenance phase.

It can be repeated if more weight reduction is desired.

Medifast, Inc® is a weight-reduction and nutrition company that produces, distributes, and sells weight-reduction and other health-related products through multi-level marketing, telemarketing, franchised weight-reduction clinics, and medical professionals. This is a meal-replacement program. It was founded in 1980 by

Dr. William Vitale, whose products were sold to other medical doctors, who in turn, prescribed them to their patients.

Medi-Weightloss® is a physician-supervised program. Medi-Weightloss providers take each patient's health profile into account when administering their products and supplements. The low-calorie, high-protein diet allows patients to lose weight quicker and makes weight reduction simpler.

HMR Weight Management® is a program designed to help a person lose weight quickly. Meals are delivered to your home. Coaches provide guidance to reach goals through weekly coaching sessions over the phone to help a person stay focused to lose weight and to assist them with adopting a healthier lifestyle.

Optifast® is a medically supervised weight-reduction program that utilizes meal replacement that transitions to self-prepared meals. It usually lasts twenty-six weeks. The program provides lifestyle education, counseling and ongoing personalized support. The process for typical Optifast patients involves three phases: an Active Weight Loss Phase, followed by a Transition Phase, followed by a Long-Term Weight Management Phase. A medical evaluation is required before anyone can participate in the program.

Some of the various methods to drop unwanted pounds quickly are described below. Some of these methods might not be a healthy way to lose weight and could cause harm to your body, or you may regain the weight you lost once you get back to your regular lifestyle as these methods are not meant to be long term. They might have unintended consequences associated with them.

A prepackaged-meal weight-reduction plan is like Jenny Craig or Medifast in that they require you to buy their pre-prepared meals. They are intended to help you learn proper portion sizes.

You should find out if the program teaches you how to select and prepare meals without purchasing their products so you can sustain your weight reduction.

Formula weight-reduction programs replace meals with a liquid drink. They tend to be balanced, containing a combination of proteins, carbohydrates, and a small amount of fat. Although using a formula weight-reduction program, such as Slimfast, will help you shed weight, it is only a short-term solution. They do not teach you how to make nourishing food choices or properly prepare healthy meals. Once you stop using the formula, the weight tends to return. I know. I used Slimfast, but failed to keep my weight off.

A fixed-menu is another strategy implemented to get rid of weight. It provides a list of all the food you'll eat. It is easy to follow because the foods are chosen for you. Unfortunately, with this type of plan, participants say you have limited food choices, it gets monotonous, and it's difficult to adhere to away from home. As with most other weight-reduction systems, it fails to teach you to make your own food choices. You will not learn the skills to keep the weight from returning.

Weight Watchers is an example of an exchange-type diet. With this approach, you have options to choose a set number of servings from different food categories, such as proteins, starches, fats, and vegetables. Within each group, foods that have approximately the same calories can be substituted and switched. For example, instead of having an egg, you could have 1/4 cup of tuna. Or, instead of a slice of bread, you could have 1/2 cup of bran cereal. The benefits of the exchange-type tactic are that it offers a variety of foods to choose from, it can easily be followed away from home, it instructs you about food selection to keep the weight off, and it can be done long-term.

It is important to choose a food plan that you can adhere to and that will teach you how to select and prepare nutritious meals so you can sustain your weight. Diets such as Atkins, the Zone, the Grapefruit diet, and others that exclude certain food groups or severely limit caloric intake may not be sustainable for any length of time. Consuming healthful and nutritious foods, combined with some form of physical activity, will help with burning fat, reducing weight, and preventing regaining it. Keep in mind that most people who have lost weight tend to put it back on again.

A question posed in a weight-reduction forum asked readers to pick which is better: diet or a lifestyle change. The results blew me away. Almost 62 percent selected diet. Twenty-eight percent indicated lifestyle change and the rest chose neither. This proved that many people don't fully comprehend the significance of a lifestyle change to being healthy. A diet is only a temporary fix to being overweight or obese, and it does not address the underlying problem of how you gained the weight to start with.

If you want to stop the yo-yo cycle of losing and re-gaining weight, you're going to have to change your eating habits, relationship with food, and your lifestyle. There is no other way around it. People who have successfully reduced weight and kept it off have one thing in common—they all modified their lifestyles and everyday behavior in some manner.

04

My Transformational Journey

You are what you eat. So, don't be fast, cheap, easy, or fake.

—Common Sense Wisdom

s with many of us, life gets in the way. I couldn't find the right balance between work, family obligations, getting healthy, or even staying healthy. I stopped exercising regularly and started eating more junk food. Before I realized it, I was overweight.

In July of 2016, my doctor told me I was in the 95th percentile for a heart attack based on my calcium blocker test. He said I had to lose weight or find a new doctor. He didn't want me to die on his shift.

In most things, I'm pleased to be in the 95th percentile—but not if it meant I was likely to die. Suddenly, my being 217 pounds was more than just embarrassing, it was lethal.

That began my journey to reduce weight quickly. I asked my doctor if he had a program to help me lose the weight. Of course, he did. Their program was administered by Cheri, who came into the examining room and explained HCG to me. She said HCG is 'Human Chorionic Gonadotropin,' a hormone produced during pregnancy to help the baby grow.

When she told me I'd get my HCG by injection, my first thought was, *I don't like needles!* I'd even have to give myself the shots.

She explained that the program had two parts. The first was very low calorie, approximately 500 calories per day. During the second part, the maintenance phase, intake increased to about 1,000 calories per day. Patients could do the low-calorie segment for three or six weeks.

I was pretty rattled by my test result, so I signed up on the spot.

At my first appointment, I found out more about HCG and learned how to give myself shots. Focusing on the details distracted me from the needles. HCG, Cheri said, tricks the body into burning fat, not muscle.

So far, so good, I thought.

"It's complicated," she said.

Ah, *there's always a catch.*

Turns out, it was more than just an extremely low-calorie-per-day diet. When people go to the extreme to lose weight by not eating, they burn muscle. That's not only dangerous (the heart is a muscle), this results in a yo-yo effect. They'll lose the weight, but they won't keep it off. HCG make the body burn fat instead of muscle.

Cheri showed me how to do the injection and had me practice. It's a simple process, and I didn't feel any pain—probably because of the extra layer of fat I carried in my belly. She then went through when, what, and how much I should eat. I was given a pocket-sized diary to record my daily food intake and hydration. Cheri said she would review my recordkeeping each week at my weigh-in to keep me accountable.

I left the doctor's office excited to start the program. Without hesitation, I followed the protocol exactly as prescribed. I made no exceptions and followed the rules. Fortunately for me, my wife was very supportive of my endeavor.

Over the next three weeks, I dropped almost twenty-five pounds. My daily routine consisted of weighing myself upon waking up, giving myself an injection of HCG, drinking two glasses of water (one with a tablespoon of apple cider vinegar), then taking a trio of Juice Plus capsules: Garden Blend (vegetables), Orchard Blend (fruits), and Vineyard Blend (berries). I would also have a cup of black coffee.

My first food intake was lunch at approximately 11:00 a.m. It consisted of about 3.5 ounces of protein (chicken, lean hamburger, white fish, shrimp, crab meat, or plain tuna), a piece of melba toast, and about a handful of mixed greens, cucumber, or spinach. My mid-afternoon snack was an apple, and dinner consisted of the same foods that I had at lunch, except I varied the protein or vegetable. I finished with an evening snack of fresh strawberries or an apple.

Throughout the day, I drank a lot of water, at least eight 8-ounce glasses. Sometimes, if I was still hungry, I ate celery or drank a glass of tomato juice. Cheri told me later that the addition of tomato juice was my doctor's modification to the plan. If I became tired or had low energy during the afternoon, I drank another cup of black coffee or green tea.

Because of my success, I decided to do another three weeks. Cheri told me that because I weighed less, it would be tougher to shed the pounds as quickly as I did at the beginning of the program.

I stuck with it. I dropped another fifteen pounds, almost forty pounds altogether. At my last weigh-in before maintenance, I asked Cheri if she thought I was going to succeed. She told me she had her doubts but was happy that I proved her wrong.

That was part of my motivation. To prove people wrong. Normally, if I tell someone I'm going to do something, I do it. I don't appreciate it when I'm pre-judged.

HCG is effective for about forty days. After that, you need to be off it for the same amount of time you've been on it. I thought maintenance would be difficult, but I actually enjoyed it, and it has altered my eating habits and how I view food.

I started each day at about 7:30 a.m. with a cup of black coffee, breakfast (two eggs and two strips of bacon), a snack of seven almonds, and an apple at 10:00 a.m. I made certain to take my Juice Plus nutritional supplements (concentrated raw food in a capsule) along with other vitamin and mineral supplements.

Lunch consisted of a protein (lean beef, shrimp, crab, lobster, chicken, tuna or other white fish) with vegetables. No bread or starch, no melba toast.

I ate my afternoon snack of a cheese stick and an apple around 2:00 p.m. Dinner was almost the same as lunch. I varied the protein and the vegetables. For dessert, I had plain Greek yogurt with fresh or frozen berries.

The trick to the entire weight-reduction program was drinking at least eight 8-ounce glasses of water each day. Generally, I drank about a gallon of water each day, and staying hydrated wasn't an issue. Usually, I had gulped down at least four 12-ounce glasses of water before 11:00 a.m. My understanding from conversations with Cheri is that most people didn't drink enough water early in the day. Instead, they waited until the afternoon and then tried to catch up. She mentioned that this sometimes acted as deterrent to achieving the results I had.

Another key factor to losing my weight and keeping it off was taking a tablespoon of apple cider vinegar in eight ounces of water each morning and drinking lemon juice. I'm not fond of drinking straight lemon juice. To compensate, I quartered a whole lemon and put it into a one-half gallon jug of water. I then drank the lemon-flavored water. Later, I found the *Smallest Juicer* in the world made by Pure Sip and squeezed a fresh lemon into the glass of water with the apple cider vinegar.

Apple cider vinegar does not reduce weight in a person who does not monitor their food intake. According to *Bragg Apple Cider Vinegar Miracle Health System* by Paul C. Bragg and Patricia Bragg, "Research from around the world supports and commends what Hippocrates found and treated his patients with in 400 B.C.—that natural, undistilled Apple Cider Vinegar (or ACV) is a powerful cleansing and healing elixir for a healthier, stronger, longer life!" The Braggs stated that apple cider vinegar has been used throughout time by many cultures including, but not limited to, the Babylonians, the Egyptians, the Greek and Romans, and in Biblical times as an antiseptic and healing agent and is mentioned in the Bible.

One reason given for the benefits of apple cider vinegar is apples are a good source of potassium. Potassium is required to build and maintain healthy tissues. Unfortunately, most humans are deficient in potassium and it's reflected in their poor health. Just recently I discovered Bragg's Organic Apple Cider Vinegar All Natural Drink, Apple-Cinnamon. It's delicious. Now I enjoy getting my daily dose of apple cider vinegar with this great tasting beverage.

For me, it was a decision to make a lifestyle change. I prefer to eat the new way. Occasionally, now that I have reached my weight goal, I will indulge and treat myself to a slice of pizza, a scoop of ice cream, a piece of candy, or a bite of bread. The difference now from before is that I have a small amount. I reduced the quantity of what I consume. I don't have two scoops of ice cream or devour an entire pizza. Instead of scarfing down four or five slices of bread, I might have a bite or two from one piece. If I can do it, you can do it too.

Another reason I had success getting rid of weight was eating slowly. With the smaller portions, I wanted to savor each bite. This was a big change for me. Before the weight-reduction program, I ate extremely fast. I'm certain many of you are thinking, *Yeah, sure, how fast can he have eaten his food?* Let me give you some examples of how fast I ate.

When I was in high school, my twin brother Larry, our friend Warren, and I sat down for lunch. My mom had just served Warren and Larry their food. My brother asked, "Aren't you going to give David his food?"

To which my mother responded, "I did. He ate it already."

I had cleaned my plate before Warren and Larry had a chance to start enjoying their meal. It wasn't that I ate my food, it was more that I inhaled it.

During my first year in college, about twice a week, a group of us played cards and ordered in pizza. Soon afterwards, my friends suspected something wasn't quite right. One evening, after all the pizza had been eaten, Paul said, "I only had one piece."

Eric also said, "I only had one slice."

Jim looked at them and said, "Hey, I only had one slice."

They all looked at me. Jim asked, "David, how many did you eat?"

Sheepishly, I replied, "I guess I had the rest." About five slices.

After that, they limited me to two slices.

During my sophomore year, I had six plates of spaghetti within ten minutes. The girl serving the food in the cafeteria asked me on the sixth serving, "Are you eating this or dumping it?"

"I'm eating it."

She just shook her head.

My nickname in college was Turbo, short for turbo charger. A fraternity brother pinned that name on me because as he put it, I ate so fast, I acted like a turbo-charged engine guzzling gas.

Despite my poor eating habits, I weighed 155 pounds. I got away with eating a lot and eating quickly because I exercised a lot. I did a special workout with light weights, push-ups, and sit-ups. Plus, I jogged about two miles each day. I burned off the extra calories.

While in college, I went with friends to a restaurant to celebrate a friend's birthday. I ordered lobster tail. To my friends' amazement, I finished my meal last, and they asked me if I was sick or felt ill.

I said, "No, I wanted to enjoy it."

The point of this is that I had the ability to eat leisurely, but I chose not to do so all other times. If you make a conscientious decision, you can eat slower. Yes, you can persuade people to change. I'm a perfect example.

You might be wondering why I choose HCG over every other weight-reduction/diet program. Simple. Because nothing else I tried worked for me. I'm the typical male who thinks he can drop weight quickly simply by exercising more and eating less. But, like many other men, I'd give up after a few days, or even, maybe a few weeks. Like so many people who promise themselves on New Years' Day to lose weight, I broke my promise. Most individuals who make a New Year's resolution to shed weight generally break that promise by mid-January, if not sooner.

I found a business card that billionaire Bill Bartmann had given to me in 2007. The purpose of the card was to write down a goal and a date that I wanted to achieve my goal by.

My goal was to weigh 165 pounds by December 31, 2008. I didn't reach that goal until November 15, 2016. It took me almost eight years to reach that weight, despite having put my desire in writing.

I read many books on weight loss. I tried Mack Newton's 3–2 Eating Plan. It had worked for so many others. Mack Newton has an awesome reputation and his clients get amazing results. I tried several ways to get rid of the extra weight, but nothing worked for me. I struggled to shed those extra unwanted pounds. Why? One factor. I didn't join Mack Newton's program. I had no one keeping me accountable.

Who's keeping you accountable? Controlling the person in the mirror is a key to success to weight reduction. It's what you do when nobody is looking that keeps you on track.

People who talk to me about HCG get turned off because they need to inject themselves every day. At first, I was apprehensive about injecting myself too. But, when Cheri showed me how to do it and had me do it myself, it was easy. You shouldn't be afraid of the needle. It is a very tiny needle. I barely felt it, if at all. Besides, you only inject yourself each day for either three or six weeks. It is only temporary.

They do offer drops of HCG instead of injections. You need to talk with your doctor about using drops. The injections have been proven to be more effective.

Another factor that turns people off the HCG program is consuming approximately 500 calories a day. When I tell people that this is how I lost the weight so quickly, their initial response is, "I can't do that," or "That can't be healthy." To me, that is a defeatist attitude. How do they know they won't be able to do it without at least trying? It's a matter of believing you can do it. I had no doubts in my mind that I was going to succeed.

As to it being healthy or not, there are mixed feelings about this issue depending on who you speak to. I did the program under a medical doctor's supervision, and being on an extremely low-calorie dietary agenda was temporary. Plus, unlike many who participate in the HCG, I got extra nutrition from the Juice Plus capsule I took each day.

Natural HCG is designed to help people lose weight quickly and safely. Notwithstanding my success, I am not recommending HCG as the best weight-reduction program for everyone. There are some drawbacks to it, and one of them is the confusion over natural vs. synthetic HCG. Be wary of synthetic HCG because it has been shown to cause extreme hair loss and other significant bad side effects. I've heard stories of several people who used synthetic HCG ending up in the hospital. Even with supervision and natural HCG, the program is not for everyone. For example, it doesn't teach you about proper nutrition or healthier eating habits. It doesn't delve into the source of weight gain or how to handle stress eating. (That's covered in more detail in Chapter Eight.)

For instance, while writing this book, I traveled to Las Vegas to meet some friends. Some had not seen me since my dramatic weight reduction. As I walked into the restaurant, they were amazed at how good I looked. Naturally, many asked what I had done. I told them I did the HCG program. To which one of the group members, Emily, said, "I'm doing that right now."

I was stunned. There was a hamburger, fries, and a pickle on the plate in front of her. Alongside the plate sat a soda.

"Wait a minute!" I blurted out. "If you're on the HCG program, why are you eating a burger and fries?"

"Well, I'm with everyone here and wanted to eat."

That made no sense to me. "If you're on HCG, you know you're not supposed to eat this stuff."

"Yeah, I know."

I looked across the table to another friend. "Hey, Jimmy, when I was here in October and we all went to the Italian/American Restaurant, did I eat like everyone else?"

Jimmy looked at Emily's plate. "No, you ordered a grilled chicken breast and a vegetable."

I turned to Emily. I really wanted to be supportive. "Look, if you're going to do the program and pay the money to do it, you'll only get results if you follow the plan. I did."

"Yeah, I need to be more disciplined."

At this point, I decided to drop the matter. Part of my Code of Honor is not to judge or put my values on others. It's not my place to lecture anyone. If they ask for my help, I'm happy to do what I can to assist them in succeeding. Otherwise, I've learned to keep my mouth shut.

Without focusing on the optimal health that will reward you for the rest of your life, your weight reduction will only be temporary.

People always ask me what I can eat on this program. Here's a summary for the curious.

Protein – Grass-fed beef or veal, chicken breast (skinless), white fish (Chilean sea bass, flounder, sole, halibut, tilapia), lobster, crab, shrimp, extra lean beef, buffalo.

Note: Vegans can get their protein from a protein shake, tofu, seitan, tempeh, or any vegan meat products that are low in carbs and low in fat.

Vegetables – Fresh or frozen is preferred. Asparagus, beet greens, cabbage, chicory, cucumbers, fennel, onions, lettuce, radishes, spinach, tomatoes, celery. (To my surprise, I wasn't allowed to have broccoli or carrots. The developer of the HCG curriculum, Dr. Albert T.W. Simeons, and other researchers' studies had determined that carrots and broccoli hinder the weight-reduction process.)

Fruit – Apples, strawberries, or grapefruit.

Spices – Salt, pepper, organic herbs.

Miscellaneous – Coffee (black), tea, Melba toast, Melba rounds, stevia, Sweet 'N Low, apple cider vinegar, lemons.

Water – one-half to one gallon of pure water per day.

For information about the HCG weight-reduction program, consult your physician.

If you decide to reduce weight, choose the weight-reduction program you believe you will stick with. No one says it will be easy. The most important thing to remember is that no matter which weight-reduction program you choose, they all require a lifestyle change. You have the power to transform yourself to what you should be, but aren't.

05

Motivation

*The fact that you aren't the weight you want
to be should be enough motivation.*

—Anthony Trucks

What will motivate you to lose weight? Each person has their own word, image, sound, or something that will trigger them to want to slim down. For my friend Barbara, the word "diabetes" scared her so much that she started a program to take off the weight. For several other friends, it was emerging heart problems.

As I mentioned earlier, my doctor telling me to either lose weight or find another doctor because he didn't want me dying on his shift triggered my decision to get serious about weight reduction. Again. The number one reason people decide to reduce weight is for health reasons.

For others, it might be wanting to look good for a special event, such as a wedding or family photo. Or, it may be not wanting to take their shirt off in a pick-up basketball game. The second most cited reason for reducing weight is to improve appearances.

My friend Gary lost forty pounds during the same time I was reducing my weight. He confided in me that he lost weight because he got tired of looking in the mirror and seeing a "fat pig." He told me he wanted to look better.

Studies have shown that fat stored around the body's mid-section, often called the spare tire, increases the risk for diabetes and heart disease, and will shorten a person's life.

The motivation to reduce weight must be impactful enough for you to not just want it, but to act, and then follow through. Are you doing it for your children? Many people lose weight because they want to see their kids or grandkids grow up. Or they want to be able to play outdoors with them. It's up to you to determine what will compel you to get rid of extra weight.

Richard Simmons, in his *Never-Say-Diet Book*, stated he became motivated to lose weight when he found a note stuck to the windshield of his car. According to Richard's book, the note read, "Fat People Die Young. Please Don't Die, – *Anonymous*." Richard goes on to write, "Everyone who loses weight is triggered off by something, and that was the something for me. Die ... I kept thinking. *Fat people die young/please don't die.* I didn't want to die."

Richard Simmons acted and became a weight-reduction guru. After forty years of helping others to lose weight, he closed his weight-reduction studio on November 20, 2016.

Another example of individuals getting inspired to skinny down was told to me by a friend who owned a high-end health club in California. Upon learning I was writing this book, he told me a story of how he sold memberships to his clientele. Often, his conversation with a potential new member went like this:

My friend would say to the member, "Would you mind holding this twenty-pound weight while we tour the facility?"

Sometimes, he'd give them a five- or ten-pound weight to hold.

"Of course," said the guest.

Ten minutes later, he'd then ask, "Do you want to put that weight down now?"

"Yes, it's getting heavy."

"Imagine carrying that extra twenty pounds with you every day. That's what being overweight does to your body. Do you want to start to lose that extra weight now?" he'd ask.

"Yes."

The clients always gave the same answer, and he'd sign them up for a membership to his health club.

For me, I didn't realize what it meant to carry fifty pounds of excess weight until after I'd lost it. For years, I'd hiked Thunderbird Mountain Preserve, a hiking trail in Glendale, Arizona. Rarely would I be able to complete the trail without stopping several times. I seemed to always be winded. Once, I even tried to do it wearing a twenty-pound vest. Not a smart decision.

After I'd lost fifty pounds, I finished the trail without stopping once. Not only that, I wasn't winded. Amazingly, I passed people in front of me. Before that, I had been the person being passed. The thought crossed my mind about wearing the twenty-pound vest. Then I thought about what my friend had told me. I decided not to wear the vest. Why would I even think of carrying an extra twenty pounds when I'd just lost fifty pounds?

If you haven't fully grasped the concept of what extra weight is doing to your body, try this simple exercise. Carry a one-gallon jug of water in each hand for as long as you can. A one-gallon jug of water weighs approximately 8.36 pounds. In other words, you're lugging almost seventeen pounds of extra weight. After you put the water jugs down, notice how much lighter you feel. If you need to lose between ten and twenty pounds, the lighter weight will be noticeable.

If you don't have a compelling reason, consider this: diseases and medical conditions associated with being overweight include, but are not limited to, Type II diabetes, heart disease, stroke, liver failure, high blood pressure, sleep apnea, osteoarthritis, certain cancers, and many more. Why wait until you get a disease or medical condition that could have been prevented simply by losing weight? Keep in mind that old cliché, "An ounce of prevention is worth a pound of cure."

Are you a procrastinator? Have you put off reducing weight because it wasn't the perfect time or you struggled with it? Each day, more people say they will start their diet tomorrow. Unfortunately, for most of them, tomorrow never comes. Many more will finally begin to exercise on Monday. Of course, when Monday rolls around, there's always an excuse for not starting. I know. I've used them.

The reality is, we are all busy. We have good intentions, but for some reason, *today* is never the perfect day to start. It's bad timing, we're having company for dinner, I'm meeting friends at a favorite restaurant. Heck, like many of you, I've justified not starting a weight-reduction program because I was going on vacation soon and thought I would wait until afterwards.

The best advice I can offer is just start a weight-reduction program. It doesn't need to be perfect. As Zig Ziglar so eloquently stated, "You don't have to be great to start, but you have to start to be great." Don't delay becoming thinner or living healthier another day. You owe it to yourself and to your family. There will never be an ideal set of circumstances.

Nike had a message that really motivated me: *Yesterday you said tomorrow.* But we all know that if we put off until tomorrow what we can do today, we are just kidding ourselves. Waiting to do something until tomorrow is another fallacy. More excuses, more justification to delay, until it might be too late. Please don't delay implementing a weight-reduction program to get thinner and healthier. Act now!

If you wait until you feel like losing weight, you'll likely never accomplish it. There is never a right moment or perfect time to start a weight reduction program. Mark Twain stated it best when he said, "Don't wait. The time will never be just right." If you do start a fat-reduction regimen, be certain you're resolved to follow through and complete it. Half-hearted efforts never produce positive results. Art Williams wasn't talking about reducing weight when he said, "I'm not telling you it's going to be easy. I'm telling you it's going to be worth it." But, the same can be said for reducing weight.

Once you've decided to commit to shedding those unwanted extra pounds and getting thinner, a role model might be beneficial to inspire you to achieve your ideal weight. There are two types of role models: a positive role model, known as promotion-focused, and a negative role model, known as prevention-focused. Positive role models motivate you to achieve success or potential pleasure. Whereas, negative role models motivate you to prevent undesirable outcomes or avoid pain.

Pain or pleasure motivates people. What type of motivation works best for you: positive or negative motivation? The first thing you need to ask yourself is: what am I most focused on, avoiding an undesirable outcome or achieving success? Do you need to be told you have a dreadful medical condition or potential for developing a devastating ailment before you'll act to shed weight? At some point, if the reward or pleasure is great enough, you'll move in that direction. If the consequences are bad enough, you'll move away.

A severely overweight person worried about their health tends to use a prevention weight-reduction motivation strategy. They need to reduce weight to stop further damage to their body. In these cases, the negative role model chosen needs to be in a situation that you could realistically find yourself sometime in the future. Look for a person who failed in shedding their weight, who made excuses, kept giving up, blamed others, or justified their failure. They are a perfect role model for what not to do.

The person motivated by prevention strategies needs to find individuals who lost weight only to regain it. This, unfortunately, is too common. Approximately seventy-five percent of those who lose weight can't keep it off.

The person motivated by positive strategies needs to learn from successful individuals who dropped weight and have maintained their weight loss. They should mimic or follow the habits these people adopted to succeed. The marketing departments for weight-reduction programs are aware of this. Every television commercial and radio advertisement tout some of their customers who succeeded with their weight-reduction programs. They all show before-and-after photos as proof it can be done.

All decisions are made to either avoid pain or gain pleasure. Any act, including a decision to reduce weight, can be analyzed this way. Studies have shown that people are more motivated to avoid pain than gain pleasure. Avoiding an unfavorable consequence, such as contracting heart disease or Type II diabetes, is more impactful and powerful than looking good in a new bathing suit or fitting into that "goal dress" hanging in the closet. Avoidance wins out every time over gratification. The perception of anguish, not necessarily the reality, drives people.

Too often, emotion wins over logic. An ounce of emotion triumphs over an ounce of reasoning every time. For instance, how many times have you looked at a piece of chocolate cake, a scoop of ice cream, or a slice of your favorite pie placed in front of you and knew you shouldn't have it? We've all experienced this. Being rational, we know we shouldn't indulge, yet we surrender to our emotion and dive in. In this example, the pleasure outweighed the consequences.

The good news is that it is possible to change your thinking to move toward the positive aspect of weight reduction. What we focus on is what we create. Therefore, it might be beneficial to focus more on what we want to create rather than what we want to avoid. As an example, we can choose to move away from being overweight and move toward being thinner and healthier. For instance, suppose you did decide to enjoy a small portion of the dessert. Rather than eat the entire piece of cake, slice of pie, or scoop of ice cream, only have a small bite or two. This can satisfy your craving and not set you too far back for the weight loss. And if you do indulge, don't beat yourself up over it. No one is perfect. Just keep going and move on.

Weight reduction is not a cure-all; it won't solve all your problems. You'll still have bad days. Some people feel let down when they become slimmer and learn that doing so has not solved all their problems. However, you'll certainly feel much better physically, have more energy, and be able to do more.

The trick is not to let your emotions lead you back to using food to make yourself feel good. Relying on food as a crutch when you're down or depressed will only make you regain those unwanted pounds.

To make extra money, I dealt craps (yes, like in the dice game) for various casino entertainment companies. Usually, after we would finish with an event at night, I had the habit of stopping at McDonald's or Jack in the Box for a late-night snack. While on the program to reduce weight, I never stopped after work to eat. Once I had reduced the weight, I certainly didn't want to put it back on again. When writing this book, a friend asked at the last minute if I could deal craps for him at an event hosted at a private home. We finished after 11:00 p.m. Driving home, I had the worst craving for a McDonald's hamburger. It was like muscle memory. My working late had triggered a past memory that was still very strong.

I resisted the urge to stop and get a hamburger. Instead, I drove straight home and made a cup of tea. If I can change bad habits into good habits, so can you. If your determination to shed those unwanted pounds and slim down is strong, and you're clear on what you want to accomplish, you'll do it. By following through, you'll have the motivating element to succeed. And most likely, you will succeed.

Jim Rohn once said, "The bigger the why, the easier the how." If you have a compelling reason or good enough purpose for losing those unwanted and unhealthy pounds, how you'll get it done will come. Remember, there are many different weight-reduction programs and not one size fits all. What will work for you will show up in your life.

For me, nothing I did to reduce weight worked until I did the HCG program. My doctor telling me I had a 95 percent chance of having a heart attack was a huge "why" for me. My other why was very simple: lose unhealthy weight or find a new doctor. I've had the same doctor for more than fifteen years and didn't want to shop around for a different one.

It's a rather simple concept. Without a why you want to lose weight, you'll be unmotivated. And without motivation, healthy weight reduction will be nearly impossible.

06

Commitment to Reducing Weight

Motivation is what gets you started.
Habit is what keeps you going.

—Jim Rohn

Without changing your mindset about weight reduction and a willingness to change your eating habits, any attempt to lose weight and keep it off will be futile. It is widely known that, more often than not, people who attempt to scale down weight fail. There are many reasons why. One is that they are not committed enough to getting rid of weight. Losing weight is hard. Staying fit and trim is hard and it never stops. Staying fat and overweight is easy, and it never stops.

John F. Kennedy, during his speech at Rice University on September 12, 1962, challenged the American people by saying:

> "We choose to go to the moon. We choose to go to the moon in this decade and do other things, not because they are easy, but because they are hard; because that

goal will serve to organize and measure the best of our energies and skills; because that challenge is one that we're willing to accept...."

You must decide if you are committed to reducing weight. Being motivated is different from being committed. Motivation will get you started, commitment will keep you going. My definition of commitment is to devote yourself universally and without reservation. Once you steadfastly commit to getting rid of weight and are resolute in your determination to do so, the universe will assist you, guide you, support you, and even create miracles for you. You just need to believe in yourself—believe that you can do it.

If I had been committed to losing weight a long time ago, I would have lost it earlier. Since results do not lie, I obviously wasn't committed to slimming down. I made excuses to justify my failure to lose weight. You either have excuses, or you have results. There is no in-between. When you stop making excuses for failing to shed your excess weight, you'll find the results you want.

To achieve long-term weight reduction, a person must make ongoing changes in their lifestyle and eating habits. Permanent weight reduction takes time, effort, and a lifelong commitment. People lose weight all the time, but most them gain it back and then some. Make sure you're ready to make everlasting changes and that you want to do it for the right reasons.

To stay committed to a weight-reduction program, you must be dedicated and determined. It takes a lot of mental and physical energy to change your lifestyle. Good routines are hard to keep. Bad habits are hard to break.

Be careful of exceptions. They tend to become the rule. I'm talking about the little voices in your head saying, "It's okay to eat that candy bar or cookie," or "You've earned that piece of pie or desert."

No! It's not okay to have that candy bar or eat a cookie. No! It's not okay to treat yourself if you're still overweight. Do you want to reduce your weight? If so, what are you willing to give up or sacrifice to make it happen? Do you really need that piece of cake? Do you need to eat that cookie or pint of ice cream? Give up what you want today so you can get what you want tomorrow.

I turned down eating what I wasn't supposed to consume to be trim. My friend Emily, whom I mentioned earlier, caved in, and had a burger with fries instead a burger without the bun or perhaps a plain grilled chicken breast. As I said, good routines are hard to keep. Bad habits are hard to break.

Have you had someone tell you, "Have just one. It won't kill you." It may not kill you, but it will keep you from achieving your goal of getting rid of weight. Be polite, but respectfully decline. The word "no" is a complete sentence. Just say, "No thank you." You don't need to give an explanation.

There are many more variations of making an exception, so be wary. There are people who will tell you, "You can't lose weight, so just go ahead and eat." Or, "You won't be able to do it. So, why bother?" Don't believe them because they are the ones that can't. I'll repeat it once more. "Be careful of exceptions. They tend to become the rule."

Sticking with your commitment is tough during the holidays. The words, "I'm on a restrictive diet," at restaurants helped me tremendously. As I stated before, it's amazing how many servers, whether it be for fast food or fine dining, want to help you succeed.

Friends or family members might react differently. Of course, they would want you to succeed with your weight-reduction program, but they might feel offended when you show up and decline the food they spent two days preparing. After all, they did go through the expense and trouble to prepare a holiday meal for you. Be resolved, but be polite. I used these words below to help me. Maybe they can help you.

"I am watching my weight. Please do not be offended if I refuse the food you offer or are serving. Please do not ask me to make an exception. Generally, I have found that exceptions become the rule. This is one reason I am on a weight-reduction program. Surely, you will sympathize with my efforts. I hope you'll understand why I must refuse whatever you have so graciously prepared. Thank you so much for your support and cooperation. It means a lot to me."

Sandra Yancey, CEO and Founder of the eWomenNetwork, said, "If you want to change what's visible, you need to change what's invisible—your mindset." Sam Milman said, "Thinking about doing something is the same as doing nothing." The same applies to reducing weight. Just thinking about reducing weight and not acting is the same as doing nothing to make it happen.

The brain is the most important part of the body for weight reduction, but it is the one area most weight-loss programs ignore or neglect. Your greatest enemy for reducing weight and shedding those unwanted pounds lives between your ears. My success to reducing weight began when I changed my mindset.

Your desire to get rid of weight is based on a combination of your thoughts, your feelings, and how those affect your eating habits and actions. Your feelings control your actions, and your actions determine your behavior, which predicts your results. Mastering your behavior is paramount to weight-reduction success.

Your actions must follow the course of what you say you're going to do. Most people will state what they want to do. Few, however, actually do what they say they will do. The cycle becomes completed when your actions drive your beliefs and vice versa.

Understanding your rapport with food is just as important as following through with actions and being able to resolve the underlying issues. This is mandatory for any weight reduction program.

Do you wonder why you are unable to shed those unwanted pounds or keep them off? Why you're not the weight you want to be? The source of the problem doesn't usually come from poor eating habits, but rather, it is based on a flawed relationship with food. It's from the way we think about food. So, the obvious answer is to change our thinking about what and how we're eating. Getting rid of the stinking thinking is easy to say, but not so easy to do.

Most people do not realize that their thoughts are negative or non-supportive. The only way to override the negative and non-supportive thinking is with positive and supportive thoughts. The Ancient Greek aphorism, "know thyself," can be applied to the way each of us views our relationship with food. Once we can understand our thinking is the root of our weight problem, then we can take the necessary steps to correct our thoughts and our mindset.

You need to create the thoughts you want about food and put them on autopilot so they become second nature and natural. If you don't learn to manage your way of thinking, you will be doomed to a life based in failure and struggle with weight issues. Your old concepts about food will keep you stuck.

It bears repeating: reducing weight is a state of mind. Be persistent in your pursuit to get rid of excess pounds because you will need to overcome obstacles. According to Vince Lombardi, "The difference between a successful person and others is not a lack of strength, not a lack of knowledge, but rather a lack of will."

Many overweight individuals tend to blame others for their problem with weight. You must be accountable for your own weight issues. Stop blaming others. Jillian Michaels says, "Don't blame anyone or anything for your situation or problems. When you do that, you are saying that you are powerless over your own life—which is utter crap. An empowering step to reclaiming your life is taking responsibility." Be accountable and responsible for your own issues. You are not powerless. Take charge of your life.

It has been said that practice makes perfect. Wrong. Practice only makes habit. Joe Montana told the story that when he played for the San Francisco 49ers, they didn't practice a play until they got it right, they practiced it until they didn't get it wrong. Let's be honest. No one is perfect. Professional athletes will always say they can get better. Vince Lombardi expressed it best when he said, "Perfection is not attainable, but if we chase perfection, we can catch excellence."

Michael Jordan, arguably the best basketball player to play the game, always strived to be better. It was that mentality that drove him to be one of the best, if not *the* best. Jordan knew that what he accomplished wasn't where it stopped. There was always room to improve.

The NBA 2017 playoffs were taking place while I was writing this book. The commentator for game four between the Cleveland Cavaliers and the Toronto Raptors mentioned that LeBron James, also arguably the best basketball player today, arrived at the stadium before any other player and went through a complete workout in preparation for the game. James habitually stays an extra forty-five minutes to an hour after practice and is the last player to leave the court. James stated, "You have to put in the work if you expect to improve your game." Likewise, if you want to reduce weight, keep it off, and achieve better health, you need to put the effort to making it happen. To maintain a healthy weight, it takes a steadfast work ethic.

One of the world's most renowned architects, Frank Lloyd Wright, designed over 1,000 structures and finished more than 500 of them. Towards the end of his career he was asked which was his favorite of all his beautiful creations. Without hesitating, he replied, "My next one."

Despite accomplishing so much, Wright recognized that he wasn't done and there was more to achieve. He comprehended the fact that even though he had tremendous success, there was something greater for him to do. This mindset and type of perspective pushed him throughout his entire career.

Too often, instead of striving to be our best, we settle for mediocrity. Is your standard to be average? Or do you want to be your best? No matter where you are starting in your weight-reduction journey, you've only begun to accomplish great things and achieve lifelong optimal health. Don't ever stop striving to be your best. You might surprise yourself as you move forward to your "next one."

There are those who think they don't have the self-control to change their eating habits. Willpower, a form of self-control, can be learned. Roy Baumeister, a scientist at Florida State University, after conducting many intensive studies on self-control and willpower, determined that willpower is a lot like a muscle that must be exercised. Like every other muscle, the more you exercise it, the stronger it gets.

Change doesn't happen just because you want it to. Each time you resist temptation you are developing greater self-control. Success breeds success. Confronting urges to deviate from your weight-reduction journey builds strength for future decision moments. As with strengthening a muscle, each time you exert control over your thoughts about food, you increase your ability to have positive supportive thoughts about your eating, thereby forming new habits to replace the unhealthy old ones.

The more you exercise your willpower, the better you become at controlling it. You can choose to think in ways that will support you in getting rid of weight instead of ways that don't. Consciousness is observing your thoughts and actions so that you can live from true decision-making in the present moment rather than being run by programming from the past. The good news is, your thought process can be re-programmed.

If you still doubt you have enough willpower to lose weight, think about it in a different way. Instead of willpower, be persistent.

For most people, willpower will give out at some time. On the other hand, if you're persistent and patient, you will ultimately succeed.

Either you control your thoughts, or they control you. Either way, it's your choice. Training and managing your own mind is the most important skill you could ever learn in terms of both happiness and success. It is doable!

Too often people give up trying to lose weight because they have unrealistic expectations. They spend a week or two eating better and exercising, but don't necessarily notice a significant weight loss. A safe and realistic weight-reduction goal for traditional programs is approximately two pounds per week (unless you are on the HCG program).

It took you a long time to accumulate the weight. Shedding it is not going to happen overnight. Weight reduction takes time and is a process. You must be patient and remain diligent. If you step on the scale and the number hasn't budged, don't give up. The pounds will come off. You might need to regroup and let go of what you've done in the past. Yesterday's gone. Focus on today for a healthier tomorrow.

To put this into perspective, if you lost one-half pound per week for an entire year, you would've lost twenty-six pounds. Losing one pound per week for an entire year would equal fifty-two pounds. Celebrate the small successes and build upon them. Each downward tick on the scale is a victory.

Darren Hardy in his book, *The Compound Effect*, gave an example about three men who grew up together and how "some small, seemingly inconsequential, positive changes" had a dramatic effect on weight. The first man, Scott, cut 125 calories from his daily diet. He also walked about a mile more than his previous routine. The second fellow, Larry, didn't make any changes and plodded along doing what he always did. The third guy, Brad, made a few bad choices. He spent more time watching television on his new big-screen set, ate more, and consumed one extra alcoholic beverage each week.

At the end of ten months, there were no noticeable differences between the three friends. However, by the twenty-fifth month, the differences were obvious and measurable. By the thirty-first month (less than three years) the transformations between the three men was extreme. Scott lost thirty-three pounds, while Brad gained almost thirty-three pounds. Scott now weighed a total of sixty-seven pounds less than Brad—just from a small, consistent change of 125 calories daily over time.

Hardy explains Brad and Larry face more significant issues because of their weight. Larry is almost exactly where he was two and a half years earlier and is bitter about it. Brad is unhappy at work and is having marital issues. Meanwhile, Scott is happy and is thriving in life.

Many people are aware of the negative health-related issues, such as heart disease, Type II diabetes, cancer, etc. associated with being overweight and obese, but do nothing to prevent it until it's too late. I know. I've been there. If it weren't for my doctor telling me I had a 95 percent chance of a heart attack, I would not have done anything to shed the extra pounds. Now my labs are normal, I have more energy, and I feel great. I feel it is my mission to make sure others don't suffer like I did and help them from contracting lifelong, disabling diseases.

Weight-reduction programs tend to be a temporary solution because they're incomplete. They don't help people change their thought process or their relationship with food. There is a lot of empirical evidence and data that demonstrates the majority of those who lose weight fail to stay lean. They gain the weight back. Failing to teach customers how to make changes in lifestyle, eating habits, and their relationship with food is one of the fatal mistakes in most weight-reduction programs. Too often a person will see an advertisement on television or on the radio promoting a weight-reduction plan. They sign up to receive the meals each month.

After they shed the pounds, they stop ordering the prepared food. Poof. Within a few months, they're back to their old habits and gain the weight back. They neglect to address the initial issue of how the weight gain occurred.

Although it is important to have a desired weight you want to achieve, reaching it is not the end goal. Keeping it off is. If you don't make a permanent change, you'll be like so many others and gain all the weight back. You cannot go back to your old eating habits and expect to keep the pounds from returning.

Too often, people who lose weight reward themselves with junk food, sweets, or comfort food. This is a huge problem. Once you reduce the weight, you shouldn't celebrate with pizza, a hot fudge sundae, or a mountain of mashed potatoes and gravy. That indulgence leads to exceptions, which lead to bad habits, and soon you're back to where you started. Instead of rewarding yourself with food, treat yourself to other things, such as a new outfit, a movie, a day trip. You get the idea. Stop associating food with rewards.

People without a support team or someone to hold them accountable tend to give up on weight-reduction programs. It is difficult to have a spouse eating pasta and desserts while trying to stick to eating healthier. I was fortunate that my wife supported my weight-reduction endeavor. It made it easier for me that she ate primarily what I did, only not to the extreme of what I was doing. Also, I had a weigh-in each week with Cheri at my doctor's office. Most people, with a few exceptions, need to have someone to check in with to keep them accountable and stay on track. If you can't find someone to join you on your weight-reduction journey, join a weight-reduction group. Having an encouraging community or one-on-one health coach is invaluable.

If you slip up, don't beat yourself up. Just get back on track and keep going. Too often, people will indulge, feel guilty, and quit. Just because you have a piece of cake, ice cream, or a piece of pie, it doesn't mean you don't have the willpower to adjust your eating habits. It takes time to change. No one is perfect. It's okay to indulge occasionally. If you don't forgive yourself, it most likely will cause you to snack more.

If you hit a weight plateau, relax. This is normal. Your body is doing exactly what it is supposed to. Weight-reduction plateaus are sometimes referred to as maintenance periods. During this phase, your body is making adjustments that are not reflected on the scale.

As your body changes because of dramatic weight reduction, so does your physiology. It's getting ready to make more progress. This takes time. While hitting a point of zero weight loss is frustrating, it is only temporary. Be persistent. You can drop the additional pounds and shrink your belly.

As you progress on your own transformational journey, be a learn-it-all, not a know-it-all. Learn as much as possible about healthy weight reduction. And keep learning!

There are powers inside each of us that, if we tap into them and use them, we can make our weight-reduction journey more successful than we can ever have imagined or dreamed we could accomplish. You can be slimmer. I'm proof that transformation is possible.

07

Eating Environment

You don't have to eat less, you just have to eat right.

—Common Sense Wisdom

Different environments call for different behavior. Learn to manage your boundaries. Just keep in mind that it's not "no" forever. It's only "no" for today. If Emily had said "no" to a hamburger, fries, pickle, and soda for lunch when she was with the group, it would make a huge impact on her weight-reduction endeavor.

Letting others know you are on a weight-reduction program helps. Until I mentioned that I used HCG to lose my weight, none of the other fellows knew Emily was attempting to lose weight. Again, it comes down to having a support team and asking others to help you. As I stated earlier, people who use Weight Watchers and Jenny Craig programs are successful because they have meetings either in person or online for their members to attend. Those who attend meetings regularly lose three times as much weight as those who don't. If you're not losing the weight you desire, maybe you should start asking, "What are those who are losing weight doing that I'm not?" and start doing what they do. Why wouldn't you study and learn what others who have successfully lost weight and kept it off have done?

One thing successful "losers" do is to change their food environment. Here's an example: The Delboeuf illusion is an optical illusion of relative size perception. It is widely known to cause people to misjudge circles of identical size when placed next to each other. The circle with more "white space" around it appears smaller.

Delboeuf illusion

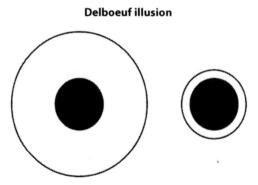

Both circles are the exact size. The illusion, however, causes people to think the circle on the right is larger because its outside circle is only slightly bigger.

Brian Wansink, Ph.D., and Koert van Ittersum, Ph.D., realized that the same applies to the plates and bowls we use every day. Their research found that large dinnerware could cause people to eat more without them realizing it because people believed they had eaten less.

Simply being aware of this phenomenon is not enough. To overcome it, the environment must be changed by replacing dinnerware. One suggestion offered by Wansink and van Ittersum is to serve healthy foods, such as fresh vegetables, in a larger plate and less healthy foods in smaller plates. Normally, it's the other way around. Salad plates are small while the main course is served on larger dishes.

I replaced our normal dinner plate with a salad plate. I ate less but felt satisfied. Using the smaller plate helped me cut down on serving sizes, thereby reducing weight.

We cannot always choose where we will be eating our meals. For instance, while traveling, it may be convenient to frequent fast food establishments, such as McDonalds, Wendy's, Burger King, or Jack in the Box. Ordering food to consume is different than ordering a meal. You can successfully eat at a fast food place if you follow certain rules.

I could stay on my diet if I ate a burger, plain and without cheese. To make it simpler for the person taking my order, I asked only for the meat and bun. This also worked well when ordering a grilled chicken sandwich. However, I only ate the meat portion and tossed the bun. I stayed away from bread.

Being completely honest with the challenges of the real world is the key to sustaining a healthy weight reduction. How many contestants on NBC's smash hit *The Biggest Loser* have lost tremendous amounts of weight only to gain it all back? Despite the attempt at behavior modification, the participants/contestants were not in the real world. They did not have to deal with life issues, work, children, financial issues, etc. They focused entirely on eating better and exercising. Plus, they had coaches and medical professionals to help them along the way. Few of us can afford private trainers or are equipped to handle everyday life without resorting to the comfort of junk food.

Foods that contain a lot of sugar, fat, chocolate, or high-fructose corn syrup are habit forming! People form addictions to it. Just ask any chocoholic. I know, because I'm a chocoholic. It's not just psychological, your body does form a real addiction to them. Dr. Jonny Bower stated in his book *Unleash Your Thin Fat Blueprint*, "Unless we acknowledge that food is a drug and that it has a drug-like hold over us, it will be next to impossible to change our addictive habits. We have to treat our relationship with food the same way as a recovering alcoholic treats his relationship with alcohol."

William Dufty, in his book *Sugar Blues*, echoed the same sentiment about sugar being addicting and habit forming. That's why so many commercial food companies, such as General Mills, Campbell's Soups, and Kellogg's, add a lot of sugar to their products. Start reading the nutritional labels on the packaging. You'll be shocked by how much sugar you are consuming, not to mention what you're really ingesting.

Many people mistakenly focus on calories and carbs when trying to lose weight. They fail to look at the grams of sugar in the foods they consume. A person eating 2,000 calories per day should only get about 50 grams of sugar. But look at what one Starbucks' Java Chip Frappuccino Coffee has for sugar—a whopping 66 grams. No wonder people have difficulty losing weight. One stop at Starbucks and you're drinking more grams of sugar in one serving than you need from all your daily food intake.

Before I decided to shed weight, I'd frequent Starbucks and have a *Venti* Iced Mocha. Wow. I had no idea it was loaded with 43 grams of sugar and 450 calories. Now I enjoy a cup of black coffee or a cup of unsweetened, freshly brewed green tea.

Do you drink soda? I can hear it now. It's only 140 calories. An 8-ounce serving of Coca Cola has 39 grams of sugar. Do you like your Hershey Bars? I did. Craved them. I rationalized it by telling myself it only had 210 calories. But look at the sugar. It has 24 grams. Just an 8-ounce can of coke and a Hershey bar gives you more grams of sugar than your daily requirements. And people wonder why there is an increase in Type II diabetes. Remember, it's the smallest changes done consistently over time that can make the biggest difference to successfully reduce weight and keep it off. Eliminating a can of soda and a candy bar can reduce your caloric intake by approximately 350 calories per day and over 60 grams of refined processed sugar.

In Darren Hardy's example of the three friends, Scott lost thirty-three pounds in two and a half years by reducing his caloric intake by 125 calories and walking an extra mile each day. Imagine how much weight you could shed just by eliminating a soda and candy bar each day.

Another challenging environment is restaurants. Resisting temptations while dining out is difficult but achievable. For example, you can win the weight-reduction battle by deciding what you will do before arriving at the restaurant. The hardest part for me was avoiding the bread. If I was hungry, I would eat four or five slices of bread before the course. Most of the time now I ask the waiter not to bring any because if it's not there, I won't eat it.

When you are out with friends, ask them to keep the bread at the opposite end of the table.

If they say, "One piece won't hurt you," remember, it will! Be polite, but respectfully decline and remind them your mission is to get rid of weight. If they are truly friends, they will understand and compliment you for sticking with your plan.

You can also still eat at a buffet if you are on a weight-reduction program. The trick is to control your portion sizes. Eating off a small-size dish can help you reduce weight.

Cruises will test your resolve. So will resorts. When my wife and I were at an all-inclusive resort in the Caribbean, the buffet became a challenge. To avoid overeating, I choose a salad plate, rather than the larger dinner plate. I only took what I wanted to eat, not what I wanted to try. When I finished my first serving, I was done. I did not go back for a second or third helping. I also declined alcoholic beverages and chose water with lemon or black coffee instead. It can be done if you are committed to getting rid of an excess of weight. Just because it's an all you can eat buffet doesn't mean you must eat it all.

For me, another key part to dining out was to tell waiters, "I'm on a restricted diet and I am limited in what I can eat." Every time, without exception, the restaurant accommodated my request to prepare the food plain, without sauces or gravy.

Being successful with any weight-reduction program takes discipline. Dwayne "The Rock" Johnson said, "All success begins with self-discipline. It starts with you." Remember, no matter where you find yourself having a meal, whether it be at your home, a friend's place, an expensive restaurant, or a fast food joint, you can make smart choices when eating if you have discipline. Getting rid of excess weight can be accomplished.

You'd be surprised how many others have succeeded. The question becomes, do you want to succeed?

Where you eat doesn't have to be limited by your weight-reduction endeavor. Little choices about what and how much and where to eat can make a significant impact on shedding weight. So, when you're dining out and are tempted to reach for that piece of fresh baked bread, ask yourself if it's worth it. Be resolved.

There's another challenging environment right in front of you. Do you realize watching television detrimentally affects eating habits which can cause obesity? Studies show a direct correlation between watching television and weight gain. People tend to snack on calorie-dense food while watching the boob tube. Studies have shown that viewers consume 65 percent more calories from snacks while watching television. Commercials displayed on the screen are prominently for food and restaurants. Viewers are inundated with subliminal messages from these ads. They're designed to tempt you to eat more, usually later at night. Eating late at night is the worst time to chow down.

The advertisements depict thin people. If you have a poor self-image, you might consume more to comfort yourself.

Television commercials provide conflicting, confusing, and misleading information about proper nutrition. Because of this, people who watch a lot of television tend to have a poorer understanding of healthy eating. One study found 34 percent of viewers were more likely to order high-fat and high-sugar foods from menus than those who didn't watch television.

So, what can you do to combat a television eating habit? One thing that I did was to do push-ups or sit-ups during commercial breaks. Start off by doing five, ten, or fifteen push-ups. Build up to a point where you can do twenty-five push-ups during each commercial break. The average one-hour long television show has between seven and ten commercial breaks. If you could do twenty-five push-ups during just four breaks, you would have done one hundred push-ups. Similarly, if you did sit-ups or leg lifts during a commercial interruption, you could do as many as one hundred sit-ups or more in one hour of television watching. Start slow and build up. Even five or ten leg lifts or sit-ups is a start and gets you off the couch.

Another benefit to doing exercise during a television commercial is that it helps keep you from snacking. Instead of going to the fridge, do your push-ups, sit-ups, or whatever isometric exercise you deem is best for you.

Sometimes, I'll lift light weights and do a set or two of presses and curls. Grab a set of light dumbbells and do some routine with them. Start out slow and increase how much you do. Gradual is better than trying to do a lot at one time, especially if you haven't exercised in a while. You don't want to be sore the next day and quit.

Five, ten, or fifteen-pound dumbbells are relatively inexpensive. Think of how much you can save by doing some exercise rather than paying for medical care that might be preventable. Better yet, grab two bottles of water or two cans of food to use instead of weights. There are inexpensive ways to accomplish the same thing.

You might consider tracking how many hours you spend watching television. It may surprise you how much time is wasted in front of the screen. Make a conscious decision to reduce the number of hours you are sitting in front of a screen.

Instead of watching the boob tube, figure out how to do something with the extra time that doesn't require being inactive or sedentary. Become active. Go for walk, hike, bike, or clean your home. Tell yourself, "I am going to do something positive to reduce my weight."

Watching television in the bedroom disrupts sleep and causes health issues. Research shows that the nighttime glow streaming from a television screen throws off biorhythms, messes with hunger signals, and has a direct correlation to weight gain. A simple solution is to either remove the culprit from the bedroom or make certain it is off before you go to sleep.

If you shop at Costco or other grocery stores, avoid the free samples. I know people who shop at Costco and other places just to eat the freebies given away. They're unaware of the many calories they are consuming. Not to mention the fat and sugars. Prior to Easter, I saw food demonstrators giving away free chocolate Easter bunnies. A line of anxious people waited to get their sugar fix, but I walked past the booth. I made a conscious choice to say, "No thank you." If I can do it, so can you. Remember, shedding unwanted pounds, and keeping them off is a lifetime commitment.

> **Did you know?**
>
> A study from the Harvard T.H. Chan School of Public Health found that people who drank two or more servings of beverages with fructose or other sugars had a 35 percent higher risk of developing heart disease, 16 percent had a greater chance of stroke, and 26 percent had a greater chance of getting Type II diabetes compared to those who had none. Carbonated sodas aren't the only culprits that contribute to heart stoke and Type II diabetes risk—so do sports drinks, sweet teas and many fruit juices.

08

Stress Makes You Fat

Nobody's going to do your life for you.
You have to do it yourself.

—Cheryl Strayed

Stress is the primary reason most people overeat. Stress is also the main reason most people take a vacation—to get away from the pressures at work or at home. And what do most people do while on vacation? They overeat and drink alcoholic beverages.

Emotional eating, sometimes referred to as comfort eating, is difficult to combat because food is used to make yourself feel better rather than to satisfy your stomach. Unfortunately, it happens a lot. Everyone comfort eats occasionally.

During my weight-reduction endeavors, I spoke with other people I knew who had done the HCG program or something similar. They all had lost at least forty pounds or more. Four out of six of these people who had lost so much weight gained it all back—and then some. It made no sense to me to put forth the time, effort, and money to get skinny only to gain back the pounds.

Every person admitted they'd reverted to their old eating habits. The main culprit: stress. If you are determined to reduce weight and permanently keep it off, you must learn to handle stress without emotional eating.

Behavior is very hard to change, even when you know you should. Chronic stress will suck the life out of you, lead to weight gain, or prevent you from reducing weight.

Stress, in small amounts, is a normal part of everyday life. Most people, however, let stress take over their lives. Stress doesn't just make you feel lousy. It's unhealthy and can lead to different medical disorders.

When you're anxious the brain activates your adrenal glands which floods your body with cortisol, a stress hormone that increases a person's appetite and makes them crave carbohydrates, sugar, and fat. Food is soothing due to the chemical changes it creates in the body. Chocolate is a perfect example. The stimulants in it make you alert or excited. Chocolate also boosts the neurotransmitters (serotonin and oxytocin) which make a person feel good, happy, or even loved.

Snack mixes, fries, cookies, and ice cream are go-to comfort foods because the high-carbs activate the brain's dopamine neuronal reward-motivated behavior. It acts similarly to an addictive drug that makes a person feel better.

Emotional eating is not always a bad thing. However, it becomes problematic when it is the primary way a person will calm and soothe themselves. Some people's eating habits are so intertwined with their emotions, they subconsciously reach for a treat whenever they're angry or stressed. I understand this dilemma because I acted in this manner. We do not realize what we are doing. You might consume junk food not because you're hungry, but because it makes you feel good. If you're the type of person who eats to make yourself feel better instead of when you're actually hungry, you need to reevaluate your relationship with food.

Overeating is an indication that something's not right. It could be anger, boredom, loneliness, anxiety, fear, or a sense of hopelessness. These negative emotions trigger comfort eating. When your first impulse is to eat candy, cookies, chips, or other junk food whenever you experience a negative emotion, it creates an unhealthy manner to deal with problems. The real feeling or issues never get addressed. Unfortunately, many people feel worse, remorseful, or guilty after emotional eating and it creates an unhealthy cycle. Some individuals further complicate the issue by binge eating. An emotional craving can never be placated. Go to the source and treat that emotion. Don't feed it.

The perception of being overweight can cause you to gain weight or prevent you from dropping it. Researchers found that thinking of yourself as being overweight can turn into a self-fulling prophecy. According to a 2015 study in the *International Journal of Obesity*, individuals who considered themselves overweight were more likely to gain weight. The study also determined that telling an overweight person to lose weight isn't helpful because it could have a contrary effect. This just causes more stress, which contributes to an overweight person maintaining their poor eating habits and patterns rather than changing.

I found this to be true for me. I knew I had to reduce weight. I had a poor self-image. But, instead of changing my eating habits, I continued to put away the chocolate-covered raisins. I ate the Pringles potato chips (an entire canister at a time). And I gained more weight. I was going in the opposite direction. Pringles for me is like alcohol to a recovering alcoholic. A recovering alcoholic should not have one drink, because if they do, they can't stop. Likewise, for me, if I have one Pringles chip, I can't stop. I've since learned that there is a chemical in Pringles that makes them addictive. Now, I avoid them completely.

But if it weren't for my doctor being blunt with me, I probably would have continued along my destructive path of stress eating. It never occurred to me that my sensitivity to being overweight caused me to gain more weight.

Major life events or the annoyances of daily life can prompt negative emotions, cause people to gain weight, or disrupt their weight-reduction efforts. Some of the culprits include and are not limited to: relationship conflicts, work stress, fatigue, financial pressure, and health issues.

For instance, a friend of mine named Susan is so miserable being married to her husband she confided in me that her only pleasure comes from eating. She gained a lot of weight over years. Susan uses food to comfort herself. The sad part is that she lost her self-esteem and doesn't care about her weight or her health.

Food can also act as a distraction. People worried about an upcoming event or stewing over a conflict may binge eat rather than deal with the painful situation.

Emotional eating provides a release from discomfort by creating a momentary sense of pleasure and satisfaction when you're confronted with something you don't want to feel. Food is a quick fix that provides comfort, companionship, and for some, passionate ecstasy. It never criticizes! It never asks for anything, and it never rejects anyone. A person binging on food because of emotions can consume an entire pint of ice cream or a full bag of chips without realizing it.

Despite the mindless eating, they may never feel satisfied once full. This often leads to more and more eating, until they're uncomfortably stuffed. Uncontrollable eating is the enemy of weight reduction.

Emotional eaters tend to eat when they're not physically hungry. They are constantly snacking because they're upset or excited about something in their life. Because they're munching all the time, they don't eat at regular mealtimes. This only makes them want to eat much more later at night.

A person who consumes real, healthy, and nourishing foods when experiencing physical hunger teaches the body that it is not in starvation mode. When in starvation mode, the body becomes efficient at storing fat and loses the ability to burn it. Eating when you're truly hungry makes you less likely to binge eat by sending a message to your body that it's safe to lose weight. Give your body what it needs, not what makes you feel better.

If you know you eat when you're lonely, plan to call a friend, go on social media, or write in a journal instead. Always carry healthy food such as almonds, a cheese stick, or a piece of fruit so you never feel you're denying yourself. Emotional eating can be your body's reaction to feeling deprived. So be disciplined and set aside time to relax and eat a healthy, nutritious meal.

Unfortunately, much like people who turn to alcohol, drugs, or tobacco for comfort, some people use food to console themselves when they're lonely. Food becomes an emotional acceptance but it doesn't address the underlying psychological problem.

If you're anxious, expend nervous energy by squeezing a stress ball or taking a brisk walk. If you're tired, rather than grab that box of cookies, treat yourself to a hot cup of tea, take a bath, light some scented candles, or wrap yourself in a warm blanket. Be kind to yourself. Self-compassion can decrease stress eating. Take a moment to think about your future. Imagine how great you'll feel once you reach your weight goal or how fantastic you'll look on vacation or at the special event you will be attending. It can help you get through the moment and resist temptation.

For those of us who compulsively snack, a great idea that works for me is to keep a cup of unsweetened green tea at hand. It's a way to keep my hands occupied and my mouth busy so I do not reach for junk food. It's also a way to stay hydrated so my body isn't telling me it wants food when it really wants water.

There are many ways to manage your stress. Do yoga, meditation, take a nap, or play sports. Close your eyes and take deep breaths. Breathe in positive thoughts and exhale the negative ones.

You don't need to take on someone else's problems. Hawk Moon, an authentic Lakota medicine man, told us at the beginning of a self-help boot camp I attended, "Your issues are not my issues. So, don't make your issues my issues." I have adopted his attitude. If a person starts to dump on me and complains too much, I use Hawk's phrase. At some point, you must let people resolve their own problems. Otherwise, it will tear you apart. You probably have enough stress in your own life.

How else can you handle stress better? One way is to increase your intake of B-complex vitamins. B vitamins are important for metabolizing food into cellular energy, maintaining proper neurological function, creating red blood cells, and more.

Everyday stress increases your daily requirement for essential B vitamins. Modern processed food is sadly lacking in vital vitamins and minerals.

Many people are unaware that they suffer from a B-complex vitamin deficiency. Over time, B vitamin deficiencies can lead to diminishing health and vitality, leaving most people feeling fatigued, stressed, and irritable.

When the body is lacking in B-complex, it results in an inability to fight stress, tension, and the strain of everyday life. Some researchers believe the excessive use of tobacco, alcohol, coffee, tea, sodas, or drugs is directly related to a B-complex deficiency.

A craving for sweets may indicate a B-complex deficiency. If you get an urge to eat candy, reach for natural, unsalted peanut butter, fresh-roasted peanuts, raw or dried nuts, oranges, or bananas as a substitute for junk food. Other foods rich in B-Complex are mushroom, avocado, grapefruit, cantaloupe, chicken, lobster, crab meat, oysters, and fresh lean hamburger.

Studies show that taking B12 can help alleviate stress and anxiety. Nicknamed the "energy vitamin," it is essential for sustaining a positive mood and proper brain function. It is the most complex of all vitamins and is responsible for a gamut of important roles in maintaining the nervous system, such as helping with concentration and mood. Because stress and anxiety have a great effect on binge eating and unhealthy overeating, it is imperative to get an adequate dose of B12.

09

Weight-Reduction Goals

If you want to do it, you'll find a way;
if not, you'll find an excuse.

—Jim Rohn

It is vital to understand that getting rid of weight is a process. There is no instantaneous solution to sustainable weight reduction. Staying slim requires making long-term changes to the way you think and feel. You must set specific, realistic, and attainable goals that can be accomplished in a timely manner. An ambition to lose as much weight as possible is neither specific nor realistic. Goals help you define what you really want: reducing weight, getting thinner, becoming healthier, or all of those.

If you have a burning desire to reduce your weight in a healthy fashion, your body can accomplish an amazing transformation. A goal is a road map that provides an explicit idea of where you want to be and a plan of action to get there. W. Edwards Deming said, "A goal without a method is nonsense." Make sure you have a method to achieve your weight-reduction goal.

Every life coach or personal trainer knows the importance of goals. They give something an aim to achieve and a way to measure it.

Individuals who have successful weight-reduction regimens take the time to create a clear plan of action. The first step is to identify your desire to reduce weight. The second step is to plan how you're going to achieve it. The third step is to measure your results along the way to determine how you're doing.

Decide your total desired weight reduction and work toward it in increments. People who are successful at getting slimmer are very clear about their intentions. Those who fail are generally vague or uncertain. For example, if you decide to reduce your overall weight by fifty pounds, set a target to lose a few pounds each week. Achieving the smaller objectives does three things:

1. Provides a systematic process.
2. Creates a sense of accomplishment.
3. Gives you small victories to celebrate.

Achieving results, no matter how small, help to keep you on course and encouraged to shed weight.

How do you eat an elephant? One bite at a time. How do you gain weight? One bite at a time. How do you lose weight? One pound at a time. Start small and create a win for yourself. When you do this, you build confidence. With confidence, you create momentum. With momentum, you take more action to move closer to your ultimate goal. Nothing sustains motivation more than a sense of accomplishment.

An excellent goal-setting approach is defined in the acronym SMART. The acronym describes the various aspects a goal should have to attain the greatest likelihood of success. The adjectives used for SMART have different variations depending on the circumstances and purpose. For weight reduction and getting slimmer, SMART is defined as

S = specific
M = measurable

A = attainable, achievable, or agreed upon

R = realistic, or reasonable

T = trackable, timely (time-based) or tangible

Be specific about your objective. Most people are not specific about a target. For example, most might state, "I want to lose weight" or "I want to exercise more." These are broad, vague statements. To be more specific, you might aim to lose two or three pounds per week and exercise thirty minutes three times per week. Your goal might be to drop two or three dress sizes or decrease your waistline by two inches. Rather than saying, "I'll eat vegetables more frequently," restate it to be: "I'll eat a minimum of one serving of veggies at lunch and one at dinner every day for the next two weeks. Clarity about reducing weight is extremely important. Your success in shrinking your waistline will be determined by how clear and genuine you are about what you truly want.

Measuring your progress frequently is as important as establishing the goal. If you can quantify your results, you can objectively determine your success. For example, a goal of eating healthier is not easily gauged. But, a target of consuming 1,200 calories per day is quantifiable. Riding your bicycle more often is not calculable. However, riding your bicycle for forty-five minutes on Monday, Wednesday, and Friday is easy to assess.

Set an attainable goal for yourself. If you have doubt about achieving your goal, you're only setting yourself up for failure. Many people claim they will exercise seven days each week. This might not be achievable if you know your work schedule won't permit it or your family obligation with the kids prevents you from exercising every day. A more manageable expectation might be working out three days each week for thirty minutes each time.

Be realistic about your expectations. Your desire to become thinner might be to achieve improved health and look better, not necessarily to become a fashion model or a bodybuilder. For most people, losing 10 to 15 percent of their body weight is realistic. The goal should be sustainable and pragmatic given your resources and time. Focus on a result you can attain with some effort. If you have a bigger goal, break it up into smaller more manageable phases. Attempting unattainable aspirations will only set you up for failure.

The goal should be either trackable, time-based, or both. If your goal is to eat 1,250 calories per day for a week, keep a food diary. Keep a record to help you evaluate your progress. Likewise, if your goal is to lose fifteen pounds in a month or two, keep track on a daily or weekly basis to track your progress. Make sure there is a specific timeframe to achieve the desired result. This provides a sense of urgency to accomplish your weight reduction by a target date.

Make a list of reasons or benefits to accomplishing your goal to reduce weight and get thinner. This is helpful to keep you engaged in the weight-reduction process. For instance, in my case, I needed to shed extra pounds to improve my overall health. This meant lowering my blood pressure, reducing my cholesterol level, preventing a heart attack, and lowering my risk of heart disease. Some people want to avoid becoming diabetic. Others don't want to take pharmaceuticals for the rest of their lives. Many older adults find that their weight is affecting their mobility.

Determining a goal but attempting to accomplish it without knowing why or without having a reason to do it is a recipe for failure. Merely wanting to reduce weight is not enough. Most overweight people want to weigh less and become slender. Acting and having goal-directed behavior is required to do so. Unfortunately, most people are unsuccessful in either starting these behavior modifications or maintaining them.

An effective behavioral modification technique, referred to as *if this, then this* process, was originated by psychologist Peter Gollwitzer. The concept is that having a specific plan for a specific situation leads to more successful behavior in handling the situation.

If this, then this helps you deal with obstacles that might hinder you in accomplishing your goal. For example, you might want to lose a certain amount of weight or weigh a certain amount by an exact date. The intention might be phrased as, "I want to weigh X." That alone is probably not enough to get you through predictable hurdles, so think about what might come up. A specific, concrete, and procedural approach might be to say, "When my friend asks me to indulge in eating a cookie with her, I will politely decline her invitation." Practice responding to any given situation you perceive as an obstacle before it occurs. Another external obstacle to achieving your goal would be if a spouse brings you chocolate or friends take you to dine out at an Italian restaurant. Do some of *if this, then that* strategizing before it happens.

Another example would be to imagine sitting in an expensive restaurant with friends. The restaurant is known for its great tasting, freshly baked bread. You love bread. But you know you shouldn't indulge if you want to reach your goal. Before going to restaurant, decide in advance not to consume the bread. Be prepared ahead of time so when the bread is brought to the table, you don't tuck the breadbasket by your left elbow and "disappear" a half-dozen slices.

Often, when my wife and I go out to eat, we instruct the waiter not to bring bread to the table. It's another way to avoid cravings and altering your behavior. Find a phrase or tactic that works for you in challenging situations.

Once you start taking action to reach your goal, you'll find that you eventually attain it. Keeping a positive attitude is important no matter how small the weight reduction or what seems to be inconsequential.

It's difficult to remain optimistic because you might feel like you're not losing weight fast enough. I know. I've been there. This means you need to deal with internal impediments–your own thoughts. Thinking "This is too hard" or "I don't have time to exercise or prepare healthy meals" thwarts many weight-reduction programs. Be on guard for your *stinking thinking*.

The body tends to gravitate toward a heavier weight. Once you reach a desired sub-goal, maintain that weight for at least three weeks before starting the weight-reduction process over again to give your body a chance to acclimate to a lower weight.

Imagine what it will feel like to reduce weight and how awesome you will look. Think forward. You can reduce weight. You can be thinner. Leave your past thinking in the past. Once you decide to transform yourself, think in ways that support your weight-reduction process instead of ways that won't.

Do Only What You Can Do

Do only what you can do. Nobody can reduce your weight for you. This is something only you can control and do for yourself. You can't pay anyone money to exercise for you. You can't pay anyone to eat healthy foods for you. Or drink enough pure water. There is no amount of money you can pay someone to do only what you can do when it comes to your weight.

10

Declarations to Reduce Weight

A huge part of losing weight is believing you can do it.

Overweight people have good intentions to take off the extra pounds, but often fail to implement them. There is evidence indicating that people who tell their friends and relatives about their commitment to shed weight are more likely to follow through and accomplish their mission. Social media is a great way to make your commitment known. However, it can be an embarrassment if you fail.

Another method to demonstrate your intentions to drop the excess baggage is with declarations: positive statements made aloud. Declarations are important in getting rid of weight because saying them out loud sends a powerful message to the subconscious mind.

Declarations are different from affirmations. An affirmation states that a goal is already happening. This might not be true for your weight-reduction, in which case, your mind will immediately dismiss this statement. Whereas, a declaration is stating the objective of doing something.

Below is a list of declarations that I used to help me lose weight.

1. I am in the process of being thin and fit.
2. I am in the process of making better food choices.
3. I choose to get rid of excess weight in a healthy manner.
4. I am in the process of being worry free, stress free, and drama free.
5. I am in the process of being an inspiration to others. If they have done it, I can do it. If I can do it, others can do it, so long as they have the want and desire to do so.
6. I act to reduce weight despite stress.
7. I act to reduce weight despite feeling hungry.
8. I avoid eating when I am stressed, nervous, or anxious, and find an alternative.
9. I am resolved to reducing weight in a healthy manner.
10. I encourage myself with positive self-talk.
11. I embrace the challenge of reducing weight. I understand it will not be easy.
12. I act despite whatever others might think or say.
13. I adopt the philosophy of "Your issues are not my issues."
14. My clothes tell me everything about being thinner.
15. I strive to become slimmer and healthier.

11

Helpful Suggestions for Healthy Weight Reduction

Succeeding with losing weight is doing your best and being honest with yourself, even when no one else is watching.

R educing weight and keeping it off is a difficult endeavor, especially with so many distractions and obstacles to overcome. Parents, especially working parents, rarely have time to experiment and find the best weight-reduction program suited for them. Sometimes we must figure it out from our mistakes and learn lessons from what's not working. Below are several suggestions to help with your weight-reduction program, or to maintain your weight.

• Breakfast: There are two schools of thought about breakfast. The first is to eat breakfast. The second is not to eat breakfast. Some qualified medical and health professionals assert that breakfast is the most important meal of the day and suggest a person have a few bites of a high-protein meal, while avoiding high-carb foods that can make your body crave carbs throughout the day.

However, according to Paul and Patricia *Bragg's book, Bragg Healthy Lifestyle*, breakfast is *not* the most important meal of the day. They recommend that a person eliminate breakfast completely. However, if a person is unable to do so, then breakfast should consist of fruit juice and/or fresh organic fruit with raw wheat germ, honey, whole grain cereal or an egg with a few slices of wheat grain toast.

- Drink lots of water: The human body is about 60 to 70 percent water. Drinking lots of pure, clean water keeps you hydrated and assists organs such as skin, intestines, and kidneys do their jobs. Water also controls hunger and cravings. When you're thirsty, drink water. The American Heart Association indicates a person drinking five to six glasses of water each day can reduce the risk of a fatal heart attack by 60 to 70 percent. Drink eight 8-ounce glasses of water each day.

  It's undisputed that if you want to reduce how much you eat at each meal, drink two glasses of water about ten to twenty minutes beforehand.

  Should you drink water during or after your meal? Like other issues about reducing weight, there are opposing views. According to Michael F. Picco, M.D. of the Mayo Clinic, "There's no concern that water will dilute the digestive juices or interfere with digestion. In fact, drinking water during or after a meal actually aids digestion." Roshi Rajapaksa, M.D. is of the same opinion. On the other hand, Vani Hardi, known as The Food Babe, believes "Drinking liquids during your meal dilutes naturally occurring digestive enzymes and stomach acids which makes it harder to breakdown food." She further advocates to wait at least an hour after your meal before drinking water. You'll need to decide which opinion is best for you.

- Sleep: Researchers have found that lack of sleep increases weight. While sleeping, your body rebuilds the neurotransmitters, like serotonin, that are associated with reduced cravings. Sleep produces hormones such as HGH (human growth hormone) that give you the ability to burn fat and increase muscle. Sleep also helps reduce stress. You need seven to nine hours of uninterrupted sleep per day. If you aren't getting enough sleep, your appetite is more likely to become out of control and you'll find yourself binge eating. A person who is sleep deprived will consume an average of an extra 550 calories per day.

• Avoid: Drinking soda and anything with high fructose corn syrup in it. Avoid foods high in fat, hormones, heavy metals, GMOs (Genetically Modified Organisms), and sugar.

Food manufacturers know consumers have become smarter about reading nutrition labels on their products, and they are doing everything to disguise sugar on the list of ingredients. Consequently, identifying sugar on food labels isn't as simple as before. Many labels refer to sugar as fructose, maltose, glucose, sucrose, and the worst of them all, high fructose corn syrup. If you see a product that has an ingredient near the beginning of the list that ends with the letters "OSE," avoid it. The food industry has an even newer trick: "evaporated cane juice." That's what sugar is! It's evaporated sugar cane juice. It's a well-known fact that consuming foods with these added sugars can lead to weight gain, obesity, and other health-related issues.

• Proportions: Keep your proportions small and eat five to six times throughout the day. People who eat only one or two meals per day tend to complain about being overweight. Infrequent food consumption causes your body to have an anti-starvation response. This occurs because the body thinks it is being starved and reacts by slowing the metabolism to conserve energy. In addition, it increases the appetite and fat-storing enzymes. More frequent meals will boost metabolism and the body's fat-burning mechanism. Keep in mind, though, you don't always have to clean your plate! If you are full, don't eat all the food served to you.

- Dental hygiene: If you are hungry, brush your teeth. It helps curb cravings.
- Late-night eating: Many clinicians recommend you don't eat after 7:00 p.m., because a surge of sugar and insulin right before bed turns off the fat-burning mechanism in your body. "Eat breakfast like a king, lunch like a prince, and dinner like a pauper" is a common quote used to remember how to eat throughout the day. American nutritionist Adelle Davis is said to have advocated this practice. If you don't eat breakfast, tweak the idea a bit to make your lunch the main meal.

A 2013 research study discussed in *The Journal of Obesity*, proved that *when* you eat your calories can have a significant impact on weight reduction.

Others, however, advocate that eating a healthy snack before bed might help you lose fat and sleep better. They argue that it's what you eat late at night that affects your weight. So, what do they suggest as a late meal or snack? Protein, such as Greek yogurt, eggs, or cottage cheese.

- Meals: When you eat, just eat. Most of us associate eating with various types of activities. We're conditioned to eat when we watch television, read, watch movies, or are in the car. Eat your meal while sitting down and take the time to enjoy it. Eat slowly.
- Routine: Eat your meals at approximately the same time every day. Small, healthy snacks throughout the day can enhance your metabolism and reduce cravings. Snack on baby carrots, an apple, or other fruits such as pears or plums. Avoid high-sugar fruit such as oranges and snacking on junk food. Instead, eat two handfuls of raw, unsalted nuts each day. Researchers have found that nuts boost a person's cognitive abilities, and keep

them mentally sharp. They also reduce bad cholesterol by almost 20 percent.

Weigh yourself at the same time every day. The best time for me is when I wake up in the morning before I do anything else such as showering, eating, or drinking anything.

- Plan ahead: Avoid eating what's randomly available. Avoid eating when you are stressed, angry, or bored.

- Self-talk: Don't beat yourself up for not losing weight. Every person attempting to get rid of weight has experienced the what-the-hell effect at some time. If you indulge, don't beat yourself up about it. Have the small treat and then get back to losing weight. Don't let a bad day turn into a bad week and a bad week turn into a bad month. Recommit to dropping weight. If you kept a journal, review it to see what worked and remind yourself how good you did. Review your strategies for avoiding or resisting indulging so you can do better the next time you're in that situation.

- Think positive: Avoid negative thoughts and feelings. Encouraging thoughts lead to uplifting feelings, upbeat emotions, and a positive effect on your body. The phrase, "Laughter is the best medicine," has merit. Motivate yourself with the promising messages, ideas, and phrases provided throughout this book. You can choose to think in ways that support losing weight instead of ways that don't. You control your thoughts, or they control you. Either way, it's your choice.

Everything in life is a lesson. Lessons can be learned from whatever happens to you. It's not how you respond when things don't go your way. Rather, it's what you do when things aren't going well that defines you. The key to weight reduction is to keep a positive attitude if you're not losing as much weight as quickly as you want or if you have a set-back. Push yourself to be a "bigger" person to get thinner.

- Sugar: Eliminate or at least reduce the amount of refined white sugar you consume. Your body responds to sugar the same way it responds to some drugs by releasing certain neurotransmitters. Unless you acknowledge that the sweet white granule has a drug-like grip over you, it will be near impossible to change your addictive habit. You must treat your relationship with sugar, and other refined junk food, in the same manner alcoholics deal with their relationship with alcohol. If you must have a sweetener in your coffee or tea, try Stevia.

  A word of caution: many brands labeled as 'Stevia' are not actually Stevia. They're a blend of sucrose, other forms of artificial sweeteners, and Stevia. It's extremely important to read the labels of the containers. I was shocked and disappointed when I went to purchase Stevia from the local grocery stores. Every grocery store's Stevia was a blend. I had to go to Sprouts to get real Stevia that wasn't a blend of other things.

- Dairy: Most people have difficulty digesting cow milk. In fact, a lot of people are unaware they are lactose intolerant. In addition to being tough to digest, cow milk is loaded with fats and sugar (lactose is an "ose" food). Vegetarians and vegans believe a person can get sufficient daily amounts of calcium from certain vegetables, such as broccoli, spinach, and kale. Many other people, however, have a different belief. An alternative is to consume products made from goat or sheep milk, or give nut milks a shot. Researcher have found these are beneficial to your health.

- Snacks: If you're hungry, eat a protein-based snack such as almonds, Greek yogurt, a hard-boiled egg, or roasted chickpeas. Protein helps satisfy you longer and increases metabolic rate. Unfortunately, most people choose snacks loaded with sugar, fat, or carbohydrates.

Be wary of protein bars. Most them are high in carbohydrates, are loaded with sugar, and have a lot of calories, upwards of 400. They are not suitable for losing weight. Compare this to fourteen almonds that have about 100 calories.

Cherries make an excellent snack. They're great finger food and the pits force you to chew them slowly. Cherries have the lowest glycemic index of all fruits and their effect on insulin is minimal.

> The glycemic index for each food indicates the speed that sugar is absorbed into the blood. The glycemic index uses a scale from 0 to 100, where 100 is pure glucose. Foods with a high glycemic index, 70 or above, release glucose rapidly and tend to inhibit weight reduction. Low glycemic foods cause a slow, steady digestion, which prevents you from getting hungry. A low glycemic rating, 50 or below, usually curtails sugar cravings and helps promote weight reduction. Foods with a rating in the mid-50s to mid-60s are considered average and deemed not to have much impact on blood sugar levels.

- High-density carbohydrates: Reduce your daily consumption of bread, pasta, rice, and cereal. High-density carbohydrates tend to cause a rapid rise in blood glucose levels, which invokes the release of insulin from the pancreas. This causes the body to stow glucose. The extra glucose is converted into and stored as fat. Also, insulin stops the body from utilizing fat as a fuel source and completely prevents fat burning. The better alternative is to increase your consumption of low-density carbs, such as broccoli, carrots, green beans, etc. You don't have to eliminate high-density carbs completely. Just reduce how much you consume.

- Blue Plate: If you can, eat your food from a blue-colored plate. Researchers have confirmed that blue is an appetite suppressant because it's not associated with cravings in the brain. Because blue-colored food is an oddity of nature and is not found in any significant quantities, except for blueberries and a few blue-potatoes from remote parts of the globe, there is no automatic appetite response to the color.

  One study that involved participants given foods altered with various food coloring demonstrated that participants lost their appetites when served food tinged with blue. Another study where participants were placed in different colored rooms found that participants in the blue room ate over 30 percent fewer calories.

  Red and yellow have the opposite effect of blue. They are appetite stimulants and increase your appetite. This could be one reason fast food restaurants like McDonald's, Subway, and Wendy's use red and yellow in their eating establishments and marketing.

- Nutrition: Take vitamin and mineral supplements. Shedding unwanted pounds is not just about food, exercise, and eating fat-free or carb-free. Are you aware that certain minerals can help weight reduction? Some of these are chromium, zinc, magnesium, potassium, and selenium.

- Accountability: Many people who have achieved sustained weight reduction believe the single most important reason for their success is that they had to be accountable to someone other than themselves. Being weighed by another person is helpful. It was extremely helpful for me to be weighed each week by Cheri at my doctor's office. My weekly meeting with Cheri also helped in my endeavors to shed the pounds. Form a group or have a partner to join you on your mission to healthy weight reduction.

- Calories: It's not only about calories. Too many people overlook grams of sugar and grams of carbohydrates. Be aware of how many grams of carbohydrates and grams of sugar you're consuming. The rule of thumb to determine the number of grams of carbs you need each day is based on a percent of your total calorie intake. Generally, your carb intake should be about 45 to 65 percent of your calories divided by four. For example, a person on 1,250 calories per day for weight reduction should get between 140 and 203 grams of carbs (1,250 × .45 ÷ 4 = 140 or 1,250 × .65 ÷ 4 = 203).

Your sugar intake should be about 10 percent of your calories divided by four. For example, a person on 1,250 calories per day for weight reduction should get approximately 31 grams of sugar from their food intake (1,250 × .1 ÷ 4 = 31.25).

So, if you're consuming 1,250 calories per day, make sure your carbs don't exceed 203 and your sugar doesn't exceed 31 grams. In other words, read labels and understand what you're putting into your body.

12

High Protein for Weight Reduction

Not understanding how certain foods affect you can be detrimental to your weight-reduction success.

Protein is the most important macronutrient for losing weight. Healthy weight reduction can be difficult with an inadequate amount of protein to help preserve lean muscle tissue, increase the number of calories to metabolize food, and help alleviate hunger. A study done by the Tel Aviv University found that a breakfast high in protein helped with weight reduction.

But not all proteins are the same.

Amino acids, small organic molecules, are the building blocks of protein. Protein is built from only twenty amino acids, each of which has its own unique chain combination. The chains of amino acids that form protein have different chemistries. Both plant and animal protein are comprised of amino acids. Very few foods in each category, however, have all twenty amino acids. Discussions about protein are really a discussion about amino acids. I provided this basic information (without getting into the science of it) just to show why people have differences of opinion about plant versus animal protein.

The three types of protein (the good, the bad, and the ugly) come from two sources, plant and animal.

Lean protein, or good protein, has approximately thirty to forty calories per ounce and 3 grams or less of fat per ounce and is derived from mostly from plants.

Seafood is an excellent source of protein because it is low in fat. So is white meat, such as skinless poultry (chicken and turkey), eggs, pork tenderloin, lean beef, whole grains, beans and legumes, seeds and nuts, and soy—although there is some controversy about the benefits versus the risk of soy.

Medium-fat protein, or bad protein, has approximately 45 to 55 calories per ounce and 5 grams of fat per ounce. High-fat protein has approximately 80 to 100 calories per ounce and 8 grams of fat per ounce.

Consuming medium-fat and high-fat protein can slow weight-reduction efforts because they have an elevated amount of trans fats or saturated fats that increase inflammation and cause belly fat. Proteins genetically engineered for use in food are considered bad or unhealthy. These proteins are laboratory-created, as well as chemically altered, and can cause damage to a person's health.

Many conflicting beliefs surround the ingestion of protein. Animal proteins are considered bad by some health experts because they believe human beings were not created to digest animal protein. Other experts dispute this argument because humans are omnivores. Some other so-called bad protein include dairy, soy beans, and isolated soy protein. Yet, other nutrition experts consider milk, cheese, yogurt, and all other dairy products, to be a good source of protein.

Everyone, however, agrees that protein derived from fast-food places such as greasy hamburgers and any form of chicken or fish deep fried in saturated oils and butter should be completely avoided.

Therefore, it is extremely important to choose lean proteins.

A study in the *American Journal of Clinical Nutrition* substantiated that eating some form of protein at the beginning of each day decreased ghrelin, also known as lenormorelin, levels. Ghrelin is a hormone produced in the gastrointestinal tract that regulates appetite and the rate of energy use.

When the stomach is empty, ghrelin is produced and interacts with the brain to increase hunger cravings. Ghrelin is the enemy to weight reduction because it creates cravings for calorie-dense food.

Protein decreases ghrelin levels, thereby decreasing hunger cravings. In other words, protein is a natural appetite suppressant. For the same number of calories, protein keeps you feeling satisfied for a longer period than carbohydrates. The reason being that carbohydrates digest quickly, whereas protein takes much longer. Adults need a minimum of 36 grams of protein per 100 pounds of body weight. Translated, this means that a person weighing 150 pounds should eat a minimum of 54 grams of protein per day.

If you fail to eat enough protein, you're more likely to feel hungry and eat more. A protein deficiency can often lead to loss of muscle mass. If you lose too much muscle, your metabolism slows. Because muscle burns a lot of calories, losing muscle means you burn fewer calories overall during the day, thereby slowing your metabolism. Leucine, an amino acid found in protein, helps protect against muscle loss while losing weight. It is important to consume plenty of protein as you shed pounds to maintain your muscle mass and to prevent your metabolism from slowing.

Another benefit of protein is that it promotes thermogenesis. Thermogenesis is a fancy word for production of heat in your body.

It can help a person lose weight. Your body burns calories to produce heat. The more heat your body generates, the more calories you'll burn off, the more weight you'll lose.

You can increase your calorie burn rate by triggering diet-induced thermogenesis. According to scientific studies, a person who consumes a high-protein diet can burn between 20 and 35 percent of the calories they eat through digestion. As an example, if you eat 1,000 calories worth of protein, your body could spend up to 350 calories just to digest them. It is extremely important to keep in mind that you replace the calories with high-protein food, and not merely increase the amount of food you consume. Otherwise, it defeats the process and you gain weight, instead of losing it.

When an individual consumes mostly protein and eliminates starches and refined sugars, the body will go into a process called ketosis. Ketosis is a normal metabolic process in which the body burns fat for energy instead of carbohydrates. When the body doesn't have enough carbohydrates from food for cells to burn as energy, the body burns fat instead.

Cutting way back on calories or carbs causes the body to use ketosis for energy. Ketosis is a state at which your body produces ketones in the liver, shifting the body's metabolism away from consuming glucose to using fat. When this happens, the body releases fat instead of storing it, and burns fat as a fuel. But that doesn't mean that the more protein you consume, the more fat you will lose. Protein still contains calories. And, if you eat too much protein, the body converts the extra protein into glycogen, which can disrupt ketosis.

For healthy people who don't have diabetes and aren't pregnant, ketosis usually kicks in after three to four days of eating less than 50 grams of carbohydrates per day.

The ketogenic diet is one weight-reduction program used to slim down. The ketogenic diet is centered on bringing the body into a state of ketosis. It advocates eating mostly fat with a bit of protein and a few carbohydrates. Your body ordinarily uses carbohydrates for energy. The premise of the ketogenic diet is if you reduce the amount of carbs in your diet, your body burns fat for energy. The fat in your body becomes fuel.

Some of the foods you're allowed to eat on a ketogenic diet include, but not are limited to: butter, heavy whipping cream, mayonnaise, avocados, nuts, and olive oil. But you're not allowed any breads, pastas, grains, or sugar. Many nutritionists vehemently oppose this type of method to lose weight, one reason being it's extreme. As with most extreme programs, you lose weight, but that doesn't mean it's healthy. Further, it's only a temporary fix and isn't sustainable.

Another downside to the ketogenic diet is ketosis can be dangerous if you don't eat enough protein and lose muscle mass. Ketosis can also have adverse effects on organs. Some other negative consequences are that the diet doesn't provide enough essential nutrients and lacks enough daily fiber for proper digestion.

There are hundreds of protein products on the market. Each brand hypes reasons theirs is the best. It is important to consider that some proteins are used for people to gain weight, such as body builders.

Many of these protein powders also contain whey. It depends on who's promoting the product as to whether they believe whey is a good source or bad source of protein. Whey is a byproduct of cheese production. In other words, it is derived from milk.

Whey protein is used as a source of amino acids. It has an abundance of branched-chain amino acids, referred to as BCAAs, which are used to accelerate protein synthesis. In addition, whey has approximately three grams of leucine per serving, an ideal threshold for protein to be synthesized. Scientific evidence has determined that proteins high in essential amino acids, BCAA, and leucine (such as whey), are associated with increased muscle mass, weight reduction, and reducing body fat. A downside of whey protein is that some people develop milk allergies from it.

I use and recommend Garden of Life Raw Fit High Protein for Weight Loss. It is dairy free (contains no whey), soy free, gluten free, and suitable for vegans. Also, it is certified USDA organic and non-GMO verified. Another personal preference of mine is Juice Plus Complete Shake Mix because it's a protein-rich drink mix that provides balanced nutrition.

13

Weight-Loss Principles

Life isn't about finding yourself. Life is about creating yourself.

—George Bernard Shaw

There are many misconceptions about weight reduction floating around the internet. A misconception is a view or opinion that is incorrect because it is based on false evidence, faulty thinking, or understanding. There are several thoughts about shedding weight that are not true or only partially true. Too many uninformed people who are trying to lose weight are being guided by the misinformed.

It is always good to question weight-loss "facts." Too often certain groups and businesses make statements about dieting and weight reduction that are untruthful, fabricated, or inaccurate. They will literally tell you anything to get you to buy their product or use their service. Believing some of them may be inhibiting you from achieving true, long-term weight-reduction goals.

There is a lot of conflicting information out there, especially about nutrition. Most likely, if you tell someone you're trying to lose weight, they'll have tips, suggestions, and ideas for you to try. Be wary. There are too many companies peddling products that don't work or methods that will not promote healthy, permanent weight-reduction.

To win the battle and control body weight you must understand the importance of closely monitoring food intake and adhering to basic weight-reduction principles. While there appears to be no single correct way to eat for weight reduction and weight maintenance, nutritionists, diet gurus, and medical professionals agree there are certain fundamentals of healthy weight reduction that apply to everyone. Understanding these weight-reduction tenets will help you avoid diet plans that break them and help you choose the specific plan best suited for you.

No matter how they are described, these standards are the core of every good weight-reduction plan/program, be it written by a dietician or a bestseller. And nobody achieves permanent weight reduction without obeying these weight-reduction laws.

1. **What you eat will affect your weight**

The average American consumes mostly animal products, processed foods, and sweets with little fruits, vegetables, and whole grains. It is nearly impossible to find a popular weight-reduction program that doesn't encourage people to consume a variety of fresh vegetables, fruits, and more balanced meals. You should eat a portion of protein with every meal because it's an extremely important component of every cell in the human body. Any easy way to get through the day is to have a protein shake for a mid-morning or mid-afternoon snack.

Drink pure water or green tea instead of drinks loaded with calories, such as soda or energy drinks. If you need an energy boost, have a cup of black coffee.

2. *When* you eat will affect your weight

Recent research has shown that when a person eats is almost as important as what they eat. People who consume calories early in the day rather than late at night tend to burn off more than people who eat late at night. A study from the University of Massachusetts found that people who regularly skipped breakfast were 4.5 times more likely to be overweight than those who ate it every morning.

Small meals eaten five or six times throughout the day is another proven way to regulate food intake and promote weight reduction or maintenance. The average American eats three large meals per day, with the largest being dinner. Based on my experience, the optimal eating schedule is to have breakfast, a mid-morning snack, lunch, mid-afternoon snack, dinner, and then a snack before 8:00 p.m. I understand that some experts advocate not eating after seven in the evening, but I usually eat dinner around 6:30. You need to vary your own eating habits based on your schedule.

3. **Self-monitoring is effective**

Paying attention to both what you eat and the portion size is an effective way to reduce caloric intake. Weighing yourself every morning is another tool of self-monitoring.

4. **Selective restrictions**

Almost every weight-reduction program has a list of forbidden foods—a unique list of foods to avoid. While most weight-reduction programs cannot succeed without restrictions, Weight Watchers is an exception. Some, however, take restrictions too far.

It is not safe to eliminate entire food groups because this can lead to nutritional imbalance. If a weight-reduction expert says that you can never eat a dessert again, be wary. To be so restrictive will set you up for a guilt complex and can lead to emotional eating. Thus, a person will most likely gain weight.

The more practical approach is to eat so-called 'forbidden foods' in moderation. Have a small portion and don't beat yourself up for enjoying it. This of course, is after you have reached your desired weight goal.

5. **Caloric density**

The concept of caloric density refers to the number of calories per unit in each food. Foods low in calorie density tend to be high in water and fiber and low in fat, such as fruit, vegetables, and lean meat. These foods allow you to eat them longer and enjoy more bites when compared to a high-calorie dense food.

Processed foods, for the most part, are calorie dense, meaning they have a lot of calories per mouthful. Foods like donuts, chocolate, butter, and bagels, and some healthy foods, such as avocados and olive oil are high in calorie density.

Caloric density is important for anyone wanting to lose weight. Research has shown that most people are inclined to eat a consistent volume of food, regardless of the number of calories it contains.

It is better to eat a cup of strawberries with only 50 calories than a donut with 195 calories. The strawberries will take longer to eat and make you fuller than the donut hole. If you want to make your calorie intake go further, before eating any food, look it up in a food database and learn its calorie density.

6. **Routine**

Healthy eating is not a one-time deal. It takes a daily, lifelong commitment. Having a routine and eating consistently improves your chances of maintaining a healthy body weight. Do your best to eat at approximately the same time each day.

7. **Change in lifestyle and eating habits**

Why are some people able to successfully lose weight, while others fail and quit after a few weeks or months? There is no definitive answer. However, motivation and commitment are main factors in successfully reducing weight and keeping it off. For instance, it seems that people motivated by a medical reason are more likely to succeed than people who are not. And, unless you are willing to make a lifetime commitment to reduce weight and keep it off, and have a strong motivation to do so, you are less likely to achieve your goals.

8. **Adequate sleep**

Lack of sleep or being sleep deprived causes the body to increase the cortisol hormone which increases a person's appetite, and thereby causes them to eat more.

In addition, if a person is not getting enough quality sleep, their metabolism will not function properly. Most people who are tired at work or have low energy will eat a bag of chips, reach for a candy bar, a donut, or other comfort food, for a quick pick-me-up.

A study done by Professor Shahrid Tahen at Well Cornell Medical College in Qatar found that as few as thirty minutes a day of sleep deprivation can cause metabolic consequences and affect weight gain. Make sure you are getting enough sleep at night.

9. **Exercise**

[Exercise? I thought you said extra fries!] With most weight-reduction programs, it is necessary to exercise. Activity involves body movement, i.e., walking, gardening, walking the dog, etc., but it's not exercise.

Exercise involves rigorous movement that increases the heart rate, the breathing rate, and sweat production. There are different types of exercises. Aerobic exercises include, but are not limited to, cycling, swimming, rowing, using a stair stepper, climbing stairs in an office building, hiking, cross-training, brisk walking, or jogging.

In addition to aerobic exercise, it is important to incorporate weight training because it retains muscle mass while burning fat, and increases your metabolism. Some experts believe you only need two thirty-minute sessions each week to obtain muscle-preserving benefits.

You should always consult with your medical professional and a professional trainer before starting any exercise or weight training program.

Avoid eating or drinking anything, except water, for at least twenty to thirty minutes after each exercise session so your metabolism remains elevated for a period afterward. This means that your body continues to burn fuel, including fat, after exercising.

Morning exercise, before breakfast, has been found to be the most beneficial. If you eat a meal immediately after exercising, your blood sugar level rises. This includes insulin secretion from the pancreas, which promotes storage of carbohydrates. You should not wait longer than thirty minutes to eat after an exercise session because cortisol will increase, which promotes muscle breakdown, and slows your metabolism.

14

Common Miconceptions

Merely wanting to lose weight is not enough.
Taking action is required. Being committed is mandatory!

One of the most asked questions is, "How much should I weigh?" or "What is my ideal weight?" Unfortunately, too many people rely on a body mass index (BMI) as a method to determine a perfect weight. Body mass index is a calculation based on a person's height in relation to their weight, but it is not a perfect measurement. Research has demonstrated errors occur in attempting to identify a normal weight range. Your ideal weight depends on several factors such as your body composition, height, age, weight, frame size, gender, bone density, body fat distribution, and muscle-to-fat ratio.

Further, BMI fails to indicate a person's healthiness and overall well-being. As an example, just because a person is thin does not mean they are healthy. A thin person might appear fit, but be ill and suffering from poor eating habits, a drug issue, or a fad diet lacking in proper nutrition; nor is it a good indicator for cardiovascular disease. *The Biggest Loser* trainer, Bob Harper, is a perfect example.

Harper suffered a heart attack while working out at his gym. But for two doctors being present, he probably wouldn't have survived.

The BMI doesn't distinguish between a couch potato and a body builder. Dr. Robert Davidson, director of the master's program in nutrition and human performance at Logan University, indicated that while BMI is good to study population obesity statistics, it should never be used for determining an individual's overall fitness. Adolphe Quetelet, the mathematician who created the formula used for the BMI, warned against using it as an indicator for an individual's health. More than fifty million Americans have been inaccurately labeled as obese or overweight based on BMI.

According to Dr. Mehmet Oz, your ideal waist size should be less than half of your height. As an example, if you're a woman whose height is 5'4", your waist size should be 32 inches. If you a man whose height is 5'8", your waist should measure 34 inches or less.

Another misconception is that eating more fresh fruits, vegetables, and berries will help reduce weight. Eating more fruits and vegetables is not a secret to losing weight nor does it guarantee dropping unwanted pounds. It is true consuming more fruits, vegetables, and berries is a key component of shedding weight. But that alone will not affect weight reduction. Several studies conducted on the impact of eating more fruits and vegetables alone found it had no impact on losing weight.

While high protein has been demonstrated to help with weight reduction, it should not, however, be the sole component of a weight-reduction program. Too many people are of the belief that a low-carb or no-carb diet is the only way to take off pounds. Studies have shown that well balanced meals are more beneficial to getting rid of excess pounds than eliminating certain food groups completely.

Eating a salad at every meal will not help you lose weight either; some salads, in fact, have more calories than a regular, balanced meal. Salad items can cause a person to consume a higher number of calories and saturated fats than they realize. For instance, many dressings are oil-based. A teaspoon of oil has 45 calories and 5 grams of fat. Other culprits are bacon, cheese, and croutons.

A better alternative is to use lemon juice or salsa as a low-calorie, low-fat dressing. Or, make your own vinaigrette with olive oil, apple cider vinegar, as well as thyme and other spices.

I've heard people tell me that it costs too much to eat healthy. Oh, really? Eating healthier doesn't have to cost a lot of money. Truth of the matter is, healthy foods are often less expensive than fast foods.

Research has shown that nutritious foods purchased from the supermarket can save consumers money. In addition, it is better for your overall health and wellness. The real issue is that these individuals do not want to make the time or effort to prepare a nutritious dish and prefer the convenience of the drive-thru window or a pre-made, ready-to-go deli dinner. Read the labels and then decide which is healthier.

Another mistaken belief is that fresh foods are healthier than frozen or canned foods. With the speed at which food is processed in the twenty-first century, frozen or canned foods provide as many nutrients as fresh ones, but at a lower cost. Read the nutrition facts label. Healthy options include low-salt veggies and fruits packed in their own juice or water without added sugar. Canned tuna packed in water is easy to store and won't break the budget.

The average fast food meal costs upwards of six dollars, sometimes closer to eight dollars. Combo or extra value meals should be avoided because they tend to have more calories than you need in one course. It is also prudent to limit the use of condiments and toppings that are high in fat, sodium, and calories, such as bacon, cheese, mayonnaise, or tartar sauce. Instead of drinking soda or sweetened beverages, sip on water. Whenever possible, choose steamed, grilled, or baked items over fried ones.

There are several weight-reduction programs stating that an individual can lose ten pounds within two weeks. This is partially true. A person can shed as much as ten pounds, or more, on a crash diet within two weeks. The problem arises if you don't adjust or modify your eating behavior and lifestyle. Once you resume your normal eating habits, the weight will return. All you will have done is deplete your body of important nutrients and burn muscle.

Skipping meals might seem like the fastest way to lose weight, but it doesn't work that way. Missing meals will not help you lose weight. When you skip meals, your body goes into starvation mode and you retain weight. Your body panics. The panic causes the body to store fat and makes it more difficult to burn off. Skipping one meal occasionally won't hurt you, but starving yourself daily will. Further, skipping a meal can lead to binging or excessive eating later. It makes you hungrier, causing you to eat more at the next meal.

Pills and fad diets do not provide lasting results and may be dangerous. Fad diets and pills marketed to lose weight are extreme and temporary. Excessive calorie restrictions can lead to loss of muscle rather than fat. If the body does not get enough energy, it will begin to breakdown muscle tissue for fuel. Muscle burns more calories than fat does. If the weight returns, it is usually fat. The fat reduces the body's ability to burn calories, thereby causing an increase in weight.

My suggestion is to concentrate more on how your clothes fit instead of what the scale reads.

Another area of misunderstanding is a serving size versus a portion. A portion is how much food you consume at one time, whereas a serving is the recommended amount you should eat. Serving sizes and portions sometimes match, sometimes they don't. Serving sizes vary from product to product.

Nutrition facts labels that appear on packaged foods tell how many calories and servings are in a container. Read the nutrition facts label to learn how many calories are in a serving. For instance, a 4-ounce can of tuna packed in water has two servings. Each serving contains 60 calories. If you eat the entire can at a meal, you're ingesting two servings or 120 calories. How much you eat is the portion.

Have you been told that eating before bed will cause you to gain weight or not make you fat? Again, this is a partial truth. Certain foods will cause you to gain weight if consumed late at night, while others can help with weight reduction. The point is to be careful when inhaling a late-night snack.

There are some health professionals and weight-reduction clinics who advocate a person doesn't need to be highly motivated to start a weight-reduction regimen. They only need to begin. This is partly accurate. To demonstrate my point, consider how many people start the New Year with a resolution to lose weight. Of those people, 80 percent or more will quit within thirty days, if not sooner. Researchers have found that those with a compelling reason to reduce weight are more successful.

To be successful reducing weight you must be determined, dedicated, and committed. It's not so much about starting to reduce weight as it is being compelled to follow through. People start diets all the time, but most don't stick with it. They give up after a few days, weeks, or months. Lack of commitment and determination is the main reason people fail to lose weight. January resolutions without a high motivation to drop those unwanted pounds are unlikely to succeed. You can be the exception. When you lose your excuses, you'll find results. Get into thinking about how to change your eating habits and the type of foods you eat. Give up some of the foods you enjoy now so you can have the smaller waist.

If you're of the opinion you need strong willpower to be successful with losing weight, you'd be wrong. There are too many factors that play a role in appetite control. Among these are stress, food addictions, cravings, and hormone regulation. Reproductive hormones, leptin, ghrelin, dopamine, along with other hormones can all have an impact on an individual's ability to suppress hunger. In addition, changing your relationship with food and how you view it can have a significant influence on weight reduction. If you consider food as fuel for your body, you'll most likely consume less than if it is used for comfort.

15

Vitamins and Minerals

Be accountable. Don't blame others for your situation.
Take responsibility for your actions. The more you do
what you say you're going to do, the more things will come true.

C an vitamins and minerals help with losing weight? Yes. While eating healthier and exercising are fundamental aspects of getting rid of unwanted pounds, providing your body with the right nutrients can make an impact.

Vitamins and minerals are micronutrients, and they play an important part in regulating metabolism and optimizing weight reduction. Getting the right nutrients into your diet is important not only to promote optimal health but also to maintain a proper weight. Some of the essential trace minerals and vitamins that significantly influence weight reduction are discussed below.

- Chromium is one of the leading minerals to help you drop excess weight. This nutrient helps to balance blood sugar and enhances the effect of insulin. It also reduces hunger and food cravings.
  Sources: Eggs, fish, liver, cacao, lean poultry, and green leafy vegetables

- Zinc assists with getting rid of body fat and building muscle. It is a powerful mineral that elevates hormonal balance. Depletion of zinc causes weight gain more often for women than men. **Sources:** Oysters, crab, lobster, beans, nuts, and whole grains
- Magnesium is important to the nervous system, blood sugar, and digestive tract. It is known to relieve sore muscles, reduce inflammation, and lower blood pressure. Research has shown that a magnesium deficiency caused partly by stress might be a contributing factor to depression and anxiety. **Sources:** Cucumbers, many nuts, all seeds, cacao, and coconuts
- Potassium is the third most plentiful mineral in the body. It plays an important role in hydration, keeps you from being bloated, and is critical for weight reduction and management. Potassium deficiency symptoms include severe headaches, heart palpitations, dehydration, and swelling of glands. **Sources:** Avocado, prunes, yogurt, spinach, almonds, sweet potato, mushrooms, potatoes, bananas, coconut water, and salmon
- Calcium is needed by the body for weight reduction because it fights fat and calms nerves. It is required for strong bones, teeth, and nerve communication. Milk is a well-known source. Calcium's calming effect on the nervous system is one of many reasons a person consumes a bowl of ice cream. But while inhaling a pint of ice cream might soothe your emotions, the fat and sugar don't help with weight reduction. There are other very good sources of calcium, and most of them have additional vitamins and minerals—and very little fat. **Sources:** Spinach, kale, broccoli, sardines, almonds, Greek yogurt, chia seeds, and blackstrap molasses
- Iron is indispensable for metabolism and weight reduction. It is an essential mineral because of its role in the synthesis of hemoglobin, which helps red blood cells carry oxygen to all the tissues

in our body. Approximately 20 percent of women and 50 percent of pregnant women are iron-deficient. Less than 3 percent of men have low iron. If you notice it's difficult to lose weight, and you're always fatigued, weak, or irritable, and are unable to stay focused, you might want to get your iron level tested. There are two types of dietary iron: heme and non-heme. Heme iron is found in foods rich in hemoglobin and myoglobin, such as fish, meat, and poultry. Non-heme is derived from fruits, vegetables, and legumes. Research indicates that Vitamin C may dramatically increase the absorption of non-heme iron.

Being overweight can hinder the absorption of iron, which then could adversely affect the thyroid, thereby leading to weight gain.

Sources: Liver (beef or chicken), clams, oysters, canned sardines, prunes, beans, apricots, and spinach

- Sulfur is one of the more abundant minerals in our bodies. It's important for the detoxification of metals and other toxins and in the nutrient transport to and from cells.

Sources: Garlic, onions, asparagus, eggs, fish, and cacao

- Selenium is a trace mineral necessary for good thyroid performance, a healthy immune system, and cognitive function. Selenium deficiency is rare. Although selenium supplements are available, it's best to get it through food.

Sources: Brazil nuts, halibut, tuna, and organ meats

- Iodine is a major component of the hormones made in the thyroid. The proper balance of iodine in the thyroid gland is delicate because either too much or too little can slow down the production of hormones that regulate metabolism.

Sources: Scallops, yogurt, shrimp, salmon, eggs, kelp, and sardines

- Copper is a key element for different body systems, such as building strong bone and tissue integrity, maintaining blood volume, and providing energy for cells. It helps with the assimilation of iron into red blood cells, preventing anemia. Symptoms of a copper deficiency often mimic those of low iron. **Sources:** Mushrooms, cashews, sunflower seeds, sesame seeds, and spinach

Vitamins and minerals do not correlate directly with weight reduction. However, they are required for overall good health and wellness. It's important to keep in mind the synergy between minerals and vitamins working together that keeps our body functioning at a high level.

16

Foods to Avoid

We are what we repeatedly do.
Excellence, then, is not an act, but a habit.

—Aristotle

When you're attempting to get thinner, every meal and every calorie counts. There are certain foods to avoid during breakfast, lunch, and dinner, and alternatives for healthier choices.

Breakfast can start your day in the right direction with your weight-reduction endeavor or it can leave you hungry and struggling to get through the rest of the day. A healthy breakfast should have 25 to 35 grams of protein, between 15 and 25 grams of healthy fat, and 8 grams of fiber from whole, unprocessed foods. A 450-calorie breakfast will help you to shed unwanted pounds. If, however, you are maintaining weight or are exercising, 550 calories are more appropriate.

A common misconception is that breakfast cereals are nutritious. They aren't. They often contain only small amounts of whole grains despite the packaging claiming otherwise. The grains are highly processed and nutrients are artificially added.

Pancakes and waffles are not better as a healthy breakfast for losing weight. Although they have more protein than many other breakfast items, they are made with refined flour. Researchers suggests that these refined grains, such as wheat flour, are inclined to cause insulin resistance and obesity. Furthermore, people usually pour pancake syrup over this starch-based batter concoction. Pancake syrup, unlike maple syrup, is made with high-fructose corn syrup. High-fructose corn syrup can cause inflammation that pushes insulin resistance, which can lead to prediabetes or Type II diabetes. Maple syrup is a better choice, but it's still high in empty calories.

Whole grain toast smeared with margarine is unhealthy because the margarine contains trans fats, which are the unhealthiest type of fats you can put into your body. There's an enormous amount of evidence that trans fats are extremely inflammatory and increase your risk of developing a disease. Whole grain toast smothered with butter isn't much better, but for different reasons: extra calories from saturated fat.

Muffins have a reputation of being a healthy breakfast choice. Most muffins are small cakes in disguise. They are made from enriched flour, sugar, and butter. Commercially sold muffins tend to be oversized and more than 300 percent larger than the USDA recommend portion. Frequently, muffins are covered with sugar or filled with chocolate chips or dried fruit, increasing the sugar and calorie count. They tend to have a high glycemic index. You might want to rethink devouring a muffin and cup of coffee for breakfast if you want to lose weight.

Oatmeal should be eaten at lunch instead of breakfast because it has high carbs. Eating a high amount of carbs early in the day will generally increase your cravings for carbohydrates through the remainder of the day. Most people add milk and sugar to oatmeal, which also adds calories. A healthier alternative is to add strawberries or blueberries to sweeten the dish.

Toaster pastries are a quick and easy breakfast option, but not a good one. For example, Pop Tarts are made with flour, brown sugar, high-fructose corn syrup, and soybean oil. They contain just a few grams of protein. Studies have shown that women who had 3 grams of protein and 40 grams of carbs for breakfast were hungrier and ate more at lunch than women who had a high-protein, low-carb breakfast.

If you are the type of person who has time constraints and grabs a granola bar for breakfast, you may as well be grabbing a candy bar. On average, they have less than 3 grams of fiber, lots of sugar, and very little protein. Many of the popular brands are made with sugar, corn syrup, or honey, and contain chocolate chips or dried fruit. The large amounts of sugar found in granola bars can raise blood sugar and insulin levels, which can lead to being overweight and developing Type II diabetes.

Eating a medium-size orange may be good for weight reduction because it averages about 45 calories and 9 grams of sugar. Orange juice, on the other hand, is detrimental to any weight-reduction plan. Although it may be a good source of nutrition, it can have upwards of 20 grams of sugar. In addition, imitation orange juice or orange flavored drinks use high-fructose corn syrup and other ingredients instead of natural juice.

Now that you have learned some of the food items to avoid for breakfast, you're probably wondering if there are any nutritious, healthy breakfast foods. Of course, there are! A cup of plain, whole-milk Greek yogurt with berries is an excellent example of a healthy breakfast. However, a container of fat-free, fruit-flavored yogurt is not. Many flavored non-fat yogurts have more sugar than a comparable scoop of ice cream. Read the nutrition labels to see what you're ingesting.

Eggs are an excellent breakfast choice depending on how they are made. I will either hard-boil eggs or cook them in olive oil. Add some fresh veggies and a strip of bacon for a healthy omelet. A fast food breakfast from the drive thru is not a healthy alternative. For example, the McDonald's adored breakfast sandwich is made with an English muffin drenched in butter, with a fried egg, Canadian bacon, and processed American cheese. It has 300 calories and a whopping 750 mg of sodium. The hash brown patty adds in another 147 calories, not to mention a cup of flavored coffee.

Probably the best breakfast to consume to lose weight is a high-protein drink or smoothie made with a banana or fresh fruit. It's quick, convenient, and nutritious. While there are many reputable and good brands of manufacturers of protein powders, my preference is the Juice Plus Complete. I also use Garden of Life's Raw Organic Fit High-Protein for Weight Loss. It has 2 grams of plant-based protein, 9 grams of fiber, live probiotics and enzymes, and a low glycemic index. It satisfies hunger, burns fat, and fights cravings.

The healthiest lunch you can eat is the one you make for yourself, and cheaper too! But bringing a lunch to work each day might not be compatible with your work schedule. Eating the right food at lunch can help you stay energized and alert throughout the afternoon.

A nutritious lunch should have 20 to 30 grams of protein, between 13 and 18 grams of healthy fat, a minimum of 8 grams of fiber from whole, unprocessed foods, and less than four grams of sugar. A 450-calorie lunchtime meal will help you shed unwanted pounds. If, however, you are maintaining weight or are exercising, 550 calories are more appropriate.

Most people realize that gulping down a burger with fries isn't going to help them lose weight. If anything, it will add to it. Deli sandwiches or sandwiches made with processed meats aren't much better. They tend to be high in sodium, fats, nitrates, and other preservatives. Most people add condiments such as mayonnaise or ketchup, which make a deli sandwich a weight-reduction killer.

Be careful of multi-grain breads. They are different from whole-grain. Whole-grain means that all components of the grain kernel (the bran, endosperm, and germ) are used. In comparison, multi-grain means that more than one type of grain comprises the flour of the bread. It generally doesn't mean that the entire kernel was used. Don't be fooled by labels that advertise that a bread is seven or twelve-grain.

Most people enjoy a slice of pizza or two for lunch. If you opt for this lunchtime favorite, you will be consuming 500 calories and 20 grams of fat. Adding a soda will add more calories and sugar. Because pizza is made with enriched flour, it can cause you to have decreased energy the rest of the day.

Many people consider energy bars as healthy. However, the typical energy bar is made with high-fructose corn syrup, sugar, enriched white flour, and saturated fats. These are all things that can create a fast increase in blood sugar, which quickly leads to an energy crash. Energy bars are frequently hyped up as a meal replacement. Like breakfast bars, they are nothing more than a candy bar in disguise and can cause you to be hungry within a short period of time.

While a smoothie may be a healthier alternative to a hamburger with fries, pizza, or a pre-packaged sandwich, they do have their drawbacks. Smoothies tend not to have much fiber. Because of the lack of fiber, even though it has a lot of calories, you won't feel full for any length of time. This can make you feel hungry again, causing you to eat more, thereby increasing your calories for the day, contributing to weight gain.

At lunchtime, try to eat foods with high protein, high fiber, and low fat. If you opt for a salad with grilled chicken or salmon, avoid the salad dressing and other fattening items. If you have a steak, don't use the A-1 or steak sauce and select broccoli or asparagus instead of a baked potato or fries.

Metabolism is at its lowest near the end of the day. Being the last meal you eat, it should be the lightest. If you have supper too close to your bedtime, it could cause you to have a difficult time falling asleep. Many nutritionists recommend eating dinner at least three hours before bedtime.

A dinnertime meal should have 25 to 35 grams of protein, between 15 and 25 grams of healthy fat, 50 to 75 grams of carbs, a minimum of 8 grams of fiber from whole, unprocessed foods, and less than 7 grams of sugar. A supper between 450 and 550 calories is optimal for weight reduction.

Meals do not need to be boring or drab. It's all about making good choices and watching portion sizes.

17

Summary of Steps to Healthy, Sustainable Weight Reduction

Don't tell me what you did yesterday or what you're going to do tomorrow, show me what you're going to do today.

This book presents lot of information on how to achieve healthy, sustainable weight reduction. Here is a summary of action steps you can take to discover your thinner self.

Step One: Make a commitment to reduce weight in a healthy manner.

Step Two: Put in writing your compelling reason(s) for wanting to become slimmer and weigh less.

Step Three: Put together a support team. Establish a Code of Honor so that your team understands and agrees to follow the rules set forth in your Code of Honor. In the absence of clear weight-reduction guidelines, people drift. They follow their own beliefs, which may or may not be accurate.

Step Four: Examine your relationship with food. Determine if there's an underlying issue for problem eating. You may want to seek professional help to resolve the issue causing emotional eating.

Step Five: Create SMART goals. Write them down.

Step Six: Decide what foods to avoid or eliminate from your dietary plan. Discuss the types of foods you like to eat and consume on a regular basis and those foods you dislike. Make a conscience effort to reduce the unhealthy items from meals.

Step Seven: Figure out how many calories will allow you to reduce weight healthfully. Read nutrition labels. Understand what you're putting into your body. Learn about protein, fats, sugars, and carbohydrates.

Step Eight: Eat slowly and enjoy your meals. Don't starve yourself. Not eating is one of the most detrimental things you can do while trying to shed pounds. It will cause, at a minimum, physical and emotional instability. Most likely it will cause you to crave junk food, your metabolism to slow down, and your body to go into starvation mode, triggering it to store fat and hold onto weight instead of losing it. Eat small portions frequently throughout the day. Adapt to eating smaller servings more often, heavier meals in the morning, and lighter meals at dinner.

Step Nine: Be accountable to someone other than yourself. Meet at least one time per week on the same day and if possible, at the same time.

Step Ten: Exercise.

Step Eleven: Celebrate small victories and accomplishments. Stay positive. If you slip up, don't stop. Keep going.

18

Success Stories

Doing your best is more important than being the best.

—Zig Ziglar

The best weight-reduction program is the one that works for you. As you will read in the stories below, motivation, preparation, and commitment were deciding factors in these great outcomes. These people are just like you. I know most of them. The ones I don't know are relatives or friends of people I do know. If they can do it, so can you!

WEIGHT WATCHERS

Aubrey Brown chose Weight Watchers to shed her pounds. Through hard work and believing in herself, Aubrey lost more than 100 pounds in two years. Audrey has a food addiction. She had days where she thought it wouldn't be possible, but she kept going a day at a time. On some days, she went a minute. This is her story.

In 2009, Aubrey was taking 17 pills a day for depression, anxiety, headaches, and fibromyalgia. Her highest weight was 263 pounds.

She tried different diets over the next three years. She told me her struggle with restrictions caused her to binge eat.

In 2012, she went through a horrible cycle of binging and purging. She quickly sought help. Her doctor worked with her and she could reduce her meds to just one pill per day. She also went through counseling to help with her self-image issues.

In 2013, Aubrey learned she was pregnant. She stopped all medication and continued to work on her depression/anxiety disorder through counseling.

There was a downside to the happy situation. "I used my pregnancy as an excuse to eat whatever I wanted," she confessed, "and by the time Oliver was born, I was up sixty pounds and I was back up to 243."

During the next year, she lost fifty-three pounds. She still didn't feel like she had control over her food, so she decided to join Weight Watchers in February 2015. With Weight Watchers, she was off all medications and has lost another forty-three pounds as of January 2017. Her goal is to lose another eighteen pounds, for a total of loss of 118 pounds.

Aubrey told me that Weight Watchers taught her she can eat the foods she loves, but in moderation. Now, she eats a lot of fruits, vegetables, and good fats. She has sugar and simple carbs on occasion and in moderation. She says she never feels like she is restricting or starving herself. She eats when she is hungry and stays away from fast food because she no longer likes the way it tastes or how she feels afterwards.

Aubrey is grateful for the people who didn't give up on her and to those who gave her the tools she needed to successfully shed her weight.

IDEAL PROTEIN

Ellie White-Stevens, a 39-year-old marketing executive, received an alarming diagnosis from her physician in 2016. She suffered from high blood pressure, inflammation of her joints and muscles, and bad cholesterol. Sound familiar? She chose to start the Ideal Protein weight-reduction program offered by Lifetime Wellness Center because of their coaching and individualized approach. They took the time to listen to her issues and needs to create a unique plan. They also taught her how to become healthy, not just lose weight.

A year later, she'd lost 130 pounds and 74 inches over all. She went from a size 24 to a size 12.

Ideal Protein puts your body in a state of ketosis. It burns the fat, not muscle. Ellie stated that with this program she felt less hungry, whereas on other programs she always felt hungry. With Ideal Protein, you select prepackaged meals along with food items along with 4 cups of low-carb vegetables, plus 8 ounces of protein each day. She also writes down, daily, the food she eats in a food journal.

Because of her weight-reduction success, some of her family members are starting the Ideal Weight program. They believe that since Ellie did it, they can too.

One of Ellie's best tips for losing weight and keeping it off included avoiding alcohol, fruit juices, and sugary sodas. As she put it, "I don't drink my calories." She walked an hour and half nearly every day and keeps up with her exercise regimen. Instead of conducting business meetings at a local Starbucks, she switched to hosting them on a walking path. She continues to learn about eating healthy foods and how certain carbs can adversely affect her weight so as not to put it back on. Ordering a meal in a restaurant during the weight reduction phase was as simple as getting a steak, no butter, and a double helping of broccoli or asparagus.

JUICE PLUS

Linda Weigland endured a life-long struggle with obesity. In 2007, Linda weighed 350 pounds. She made the decision to have weight-reduction surgery. To get the extra nutrition she needed, her surgeon required his patients to consume concentrated fruits, vegetables, and berries in a capsule through a product called Juice Plus.

Linda said she understood that surgery was only one tool for weight reduction and that she had to make a lifestyle change to sustain the weight reduction. One of the changes she made was to add Juice Plus capsules and a complete plant-based protein powder to her daily dietary intake. She only drinks water after her morning cup of coffee.

She lost 180 pounds, and has kept it off for more than ten years. Recently, she lost another twenty pounds and reached her total weight goal of shedding 200 pounds.

Linda attributes her healthy lifestyle success to the metabolic reprogramming done through flooding her body with the whole food nutrition her body craves and needs with Juice Plus products. She says she became a part of the mission of inspiring healthy living so others can achieve their healthy living goals and enjoy the life they want.

If she notices the scale moving in an upward direction, she adds more whole foods and plant-based protein shakes as a meal replacement to keep the weight (fat) off. Linda also exercises regularly as a lifestyle change to keep fit and maintain her slimmer self.

HCG

Cheri Henry chose the HCG program to reduce her weight because her blood pressure was so high she was at risk of a stroke. The doctor for whom she worked told her she had to lose weight to correct her medical situation. This is her story.

Cheri stated she went to her primary care doctor for a second opinion. He told her the same thing, that she needed to lose weight. Her motivation to shed weight was to avoid having a stroke.

She chose the HCG program because she was coaching patients who participated in the HCG program and had seen how well it worked.

Things that worked for her were to prepare several meals in advance so all she had to do was warm them up and eat them at the scheduled times. She also drank a lot of water. To curb her appetite and hunger cravings, she drank tomato juice. To avoid temptation of deviating from the program, she removed all of junk food from her home.

Her husband stepped up to help her succeed and did all the cooking for her family.

She met her weight-reduction goal and is pleased to say that she has kept the weight off for more than four years now.

NOTE TO READERS: If you'd like to read or hear about more inspiring stories of people who have successfully lost weight, watch television commercials for Nutrisystem, Weight Watchers, or Jenny Craig. There are plenty of them.

The only success story that truly matters is your own. So, write your own weight-reduction success story and insert it here. Yours will be the next success in this book.

Here are sample questions to assist you in writing your own weight-reduction success story. You don't have to wait until you've finished a program. Doing this now as an envisioning exercise might just help you get motivated enough to start a weight-reduction program and be committed enough to stick with it.

1. What was your starting weight? _____ Current weight? _____
2. What was the compelling moment or reason that motivated you to reduce the extra weight you had gained?
3. What program did you use?
4. Why did you choose that program instead of some of the others?

5. What did you like best about the program?
6. What was your biggest obstacle to overcome during the weight-reduction process?
7. What did you struggle with the most?
8. What tips or advice do you have for others who might want to or need to lose weight?
9. Did you have the support of family, colleagues, and friends?
10. What challenges, if any, do you face now to keep the weight off?
11. What did you learn that surprised you the most about healthy weight reduction and fitness that you didn't know before you started your fitness journey?
12. What would you say to someone who needs to lose weight but hasn't made the commitment to do so or initiate action?

Have you heard these statements or similar ones on television commercials? "I lost 120 pounds on____. It was easy. You just eat the food and lose the weight."

"I lost 50 pounds on _____." I'm sure you have.

But what they don't tell you is: what did they learn? Just eating prepared meals is not sufficient. Are you going to continue to eat prepared meals the rest of your life?

Maybe.

I know a few individuals that do exactly that. They refuse to prepare meals for their spouses. They refuse to eat anything prepared by anyone else. They bring their commercially prepared meals where ever they go. They are lifetime customers to the weight-reduction company. Doesn't sound like much fun.

It's so important to learn about proper nutrition and being able to prepare your own healthy and nutritious meals with fresh vegetables, fruits, and berries. It will probably taste a heck of a lot better too.

19

Final Comments

Happiness is not being pained in body or troubled in mind.

—Thomas Jefferson

If you're serious about reducing weight, you need to be completely honest with yourself with what you're eating, when you eat, and why.

I've said it so often in this book, and I'll repeat myself: reducing weight is hard. But people do it. I did it. I want you to do it too.

Here are several keys that helped me safely reduce weight and keep it off. These steps changed my life. And, saved my life.

- A tablespoon of apple cider vinegar in eight ounces of water
- Staying hydrated by drinking plenty of water
- Drinking lemon juice
- Taking Juice Plus daily
- Eating slowly
- Drinking tomato juice and eating celery sticks as a snack when I am hungry
- Using a journal and tracking my weight daily

- Eating smaller portions
- Taking brisk walks to burn calories
- Being accountable to someone for my actions

BE HAPPY!

Happiness is getting on the scale and seeing results.

Happiness is putting on a pair of pants and realizing they are too big.

Happiness is getting great results on lab blood tests.

Happiness is having excellent blood pressure without medication.

Happiness is being able to participate in activities with kids or friends without getting tired.

Happiness is being able to focus on work without stress eating.

Happiness is making changes to my eating habits and lifestyle.

Happiness is changing my relationship with food.

Happiness is inspiring healthy living to others.

Add your own reasons for happiness:

1.
2.
3.
4.

JUICE PLUS

Please consider Juice Plus, the best kept secret for whole food based nutrition, in conjunction with your healthy weight-reduction endeavor. My mission is to help as many of you achieve good health as I can. When I was on my weight-reduction program, I fell in love with Juice Plus. I thought it was so valuable in my journey that I became an affiliate, so please pardon my fervor.

I credit Juice Plus with helping me stay on my approximately 550 calories a day while doing HCG injections. I believe I was successful in dropping as much weight as quickly as I did because of the whole food nutrition I obtained from taking the Juice Plus capsules. Unlike old-fashioned vitamin supplements, Juice Plus provides whole food based nutrition from a wide assortment of nutritious fruits, vegetables, and berries. Below are just a few reasons to consider Juice Plus with your weight-reduction journey:

- Juice Plus capsules are actual food with a nutrition label, not a vitamin with a supplement label.
- Juice Plus is the most clinically researched product done by **independent** third parties.
- Concentrated whole food based nutrition with a wide spectrum of phytonutrients.
- Recommended by a growing number of doctors around the world.
- It will work with any other weight-reduction program you might choose, i.e., Weight Watchers, Jenny Craig, Nutrisystem, etc.
- Gives you an advantage for weight reduction others don't have.

I strongly encourage you to check out the Shred 10 Weight Loss Program from Juice Plus.

If you want to learn more you can contact me at (602) 721-5218, email: **david@dbmedansky.com** or visit **dmedansky.juiceplus.com**.

20

Beyond Losing Weight

Make sure your worst enemy doesn't live between your own two ears.

—Laird Hamilton

Once you have reached your goal and have lost the weight you wanted to get rid of, the good news is, you don't have to deny or deprive yourself of everything. You can have a small piece of cake or pie. You can indulge and have a small scoop of ice cream or gelato—just omit the toppings and do not splurge every day.

Moderation and portion size are the keys to enjoying a treat but still maintaining your weight. You've worked too hard and long to end up gaining it back, so be careful. Treats can be a slippery slope. Once you start, it might be difficult to stop. I've said it before and I'll say it again, exceptions tend to become the rule.

This might seem odd, but I highly recommend reading *The Traveler's Gift: The Seven Decisions that Determine Personal Success* by Andy Andrew. Although it has nothing to do with reducing weight, it changed my attitude and my life. I also encourage you to read the sequel, *The Seven Decisions: Understanding the Keys to Personal Success* which is a revised and repackaged version of *Mastering the Seven Decisions*. Both books impart invaluable lessons about life and the decisions we make.

Reducing your weight will be hard enough. Keeping it off will be harder. The techniques you'll use to shed your unwanted pounds aren't necessarily the same as those that will help you discover your thinner self. Beyond losing weight is what you do after you've achieved your desired weight. First, celebrate. But, skip the hot fudge sundae. Instead, indulge and buy that body-hugging dress you've been hoping to fit into. Don't fall into the trap of rewarding yourself with food you haven't been allowed to eat. If you do, you're likely to return to your old, poor eating habits.

To maintain your desired weight, continue to eat healthier foods and exercise. Remind yourself why you initially lost the weight and why it's important for you to keep it off. For me, I continue to weigh myself daily. While it may not be necessary for you to weigh yourself each day, you don't want to go more than a week without doing so. If you avoid the scale for too long, you might be surprised that you've gained back five pounds or more.

The weight-loss industry is full of "before/after" stories. Rather than thinking in terms of "before" and "after", think of your success story as "before" and "now," because you're never truly done. Keep in mind, weight maintenance requires a permanent lifestyle change.

While doing research for this book, I came across The National Weight Control Registry (NWCR). The NWCR is a research group that gathers data from people who have lost at least thirty pounds and kept if off for one year or longer. Information about The National Weight Control Registry can be found at **www.nwcr.ws.** Individuals who join the NWCR are sent detailed questionnaires and annual surveys to study the behavioral and psychological characteristics of those people who have kept their weight off.

In addition, they assess the tactics being used to maintain their weight reduction.

I'd like to hear about your weight-reduction accomplishment. The stories of people losing weight and keeping it off are as diverse and inspiring as the individuals themselves. As such, BeyondLosingWeight.com is a website with tips and information to assist you in keeping your weight off. In the future, it is my intention to post stories there of successful people to inspire and motivate others.

I wish you nothing but much success.

Did you know?

- The National Weight Control Registry (NWCR) tracks people who have successfully lost weight (at least thirty pounds) and kept that weight loss for a minimum of one year. The average weight reduction for people in the registry is sixty-six pounds. Those on the list who lost significant amounts of weight did it in various ways; 45 percent said they followed diets on their own, 55 percent said they followed a structural weight reduction program (98 percent modified their diet in some form); 94 percent increased their physical activity—the most popular form being walking.
- People who have successfully lost weight and kept it off have one thing in common—they all modified their lifestyles and everyday behavior in some manner.
- When those who successfully lost weight and kept it off were asked what they did, the majority said they ate breakfast daily, weighed themselves at least once per week, watched fewer than ten hours of television per week and exercised about an hour each day.

- What's interesting is that NWCR researchers noticed that people with long-term weight loss success tended to be motivated by something other than a slimmer waist, such as better health or a desire to live a longer life or spend more time actively involved with loved ones, like their kids and grandkids.

- Most of the people studied by the NWCR said they had failed shedding weight several times before they were able to keep it off for good. Because they were highly motivated, they kept trying different things until they found something that worked for them.

- Reducing weight is hard. If anyone tells you it's easy, run the other way. But it's entirely possible, and when people like myself do it, our lives are changed for the better.

- According to the NWCR, of the 10,000 real-life biggest losers, no two people lost weight in the same way.

A1

Declarations to Reduce Weight

1. I am in the process of being thin and fit.
2. I am in the process of making better food choices.
3. I choose to get rid of weight.
4. I am in the process of being worry free, stress free, and drama free.
5. I am in the process of being an inspiration to others. If they have done it, I can do it. If I can do it, others can do it, so long as they have the want and desire to do so.
6. I act to reduce weight despite stress.
7. I act to reduce weight despite feeling hungry.
8. I avoid eating when I am stressed, nervous, anxious, or bored and find an alternative.
9. I am resolved to reducing weight in a healthy manner.
10. I encourage myself with positive self-talk.
11. I embrace the challenge of reducing weight. I understand it will not be easy.
12. I act despite what others might think or say.
13. I adopt the philosophy, "Your issues are not my issues."
14. My clothes tell me everything about being thinner.

A2

Sample Weight-Reduction Code of Honor

Below is a sample of a Weight-Reduction Code of Honor. It is my Code of Honor. You can choose which rules you want to adopt as your own or create your own.

1. Mission. The mission I have chosen is to reduce weight and to keep it off!
2. Be accountable.
3. Record everything in a daily journal.
4. Commit to learning about nutrition and better eating habits.
5. Commit to a lifestyle change.
6. Motivate, Encourage, and Empower others to reduce weight, but only if they have a desire to do so.
7. Never impose my standards on anyone else.
8. Never blame others for my failures. I will take 100 percent responsibility for my own success. No justifications! I'll either have excuses or results.
9. Be willing to be "called out" if I violate the code. My team must be willing to enforce the code.

10. Never judge or pre-judge others.
11. Do not seek sympathy or acknowledgement. I want to reduce weight and keep it off for me. Not anyone else. No one can do it for me. I must be willing to do it myself.

Agreed to by: _____

A3

Recommended Books

Bragg Healthy Lifestyle, Vital Living to 120! by Paul and Patricia Bragg (and all the other books written by Paul and Patricia Bragg)

Sugar Blues by William Dufty

Fountain of Youth by Peter Kelder

Never-Say-Diet Book by Richard Simmons

The Maker's Diet by Jordan Rubin

Perfect Weight by Jordan Rubin

Unleash Your Thin Fat Burning Blueprint by Jonny Bowden, PhD

Forks Over Knives, The Plant-Based Way to Health by Del Sroufe and Chandra Moskowitz

The Biggest Loser, The Weight-Loss Program to Transform Your Body, Health, and Life—Adapted from NBC's Hit Show! by Maggie Greenwood-Robinson and Cheryl Forberg

The Biggest Loser Cookbook by Devin Alexander and Karen Kaplan

The Blue Zones by Dan Buettner

The Traveler's Gift by Andy Andrews

The Plant Paradox, The Hidden Dangers in "Healthy" Foods That Cause Disease and Weight Gain by Steven R. Gundry, MD

NOTE TO READERS: I have read the books listed above throughout my life. Go to any bookstore and you will see hundreds and hundreds of diet and weight-loss books. You need to figure out which book(s) are right for you. To determine which books are right for you, ask people you trust for recommendations, or check out reviews on Amazon.

A4

Contact Information for Weight Reduction Programs

Curves/Jenny Craig: Telephone: 866-706-4042
Website: **www.jennycraig.com**

Weight Watchers: Website: **www.weightwatchers.com**

Juice Plus: Telephone 1-602-721-5218
Websites: **www.dmedansky.juiceplus.com**

Ideal Protein: Telephone: 1-866-314-4447
Website: **www.idealprotein.com**

Nutrisystem: Telephone: 1-888-675-7525
Website: **www.nutrisystem.com**

Medifast, Inc.: Telephone: 1-800-209-0878
Website: **www.medfast1.com**

Medi-Weightloss: Telephone: 1-877-MED-LOSS
Website: **www.mediweightloss.com**

HMR Weight
Management:
Telephone: 877-501-7833 or
800-648-1632
Website: **www.hmrprogram.com**

A5

Example of a Weight-Reduction Diary Sheet

There may be times when you have food, drinks, or activities (both work or play) that might affect your amount of weight reduction. A properly completed diary is the ideal tool to help you identify the issue. Be accountable. Record everything accurately.

Date: Weight: Daily Change: _____   Total Pounds Lost _____

Water (8 oz. glasses): √   √   __ __ __ __ __ __ __ __
              1   2   3   4   5   6   7   8   9   10

BREAKFAST:
Two Eggs: 148, *2 strips Bacon*: 86, *whole Banana*: 105, *two Dates*: 70 each

10:00 A.M. SNACK: *Apple*: 95, *Almonds (7)*: 55

LUNCH:
Protein: *Hamburger*: 130/patty, or *Chicken Breast*: 187/4.5 oz.
Fruit: *Pear*: 102
Vegetable: *Avocado*: 114/half, or ½ cup *Baby Carrots*: 4 each
Starch: _____
2:00 P.M. SNACK: *Cheese stick*: 80, *Apple*: 95, or *Pear*: 102

DISCOVER YOUR THINNER SELF

DINNER:

Protein: *Ravioli*: 230/serving, or *Salmon*: 207/4 oz.

Fruit: _____

Vegetable: ½ cup *Cabbage*: 15, or *Cucumbe*r: 8/½ cup, or *Peas*: 118/cup

Starch: _____

7:00 P.M. SNACK: *Greek Yogurt (Individual serving)*: 100, *Blueberries*: 85/cup

Daily Miscellaneous: *Apple Cider Vinegar* – 1 tbsp. *Lemon Juice*

NOTE: If you choose to do so, you can calculate how many calories you've eaten each day. But, it is not necessary. If I start to gain weight, I determine if I am consuming too many calories to get back on track.

I have a list of the foods I eat with the calories for each for a quick reference. Make your own list based on your food preferences.

A6

Foods to Avoid to Help Reduce Weight

B elow is only a partial list of foods to avoid when you are on a weight-reduction program. Once you have reached your desired weight goal, they all may be consumed in moderation.

1. Potatoes
2. Rice, wheat, or other grains (peas and corn) and starches
3. Pasta
4. Cereal
5. Bread
6. Sugar
7. Alcohol
8. Dairy
9. Fruit (Exception: you should eat at least one apple per day. If you don't like apples, one-half grapefruit or one-half cup of berries is okay).
10. Candy
11. Soda
12. Pastries

13. Potato chips or French fries or tortilla chips
14. Pancakes or waffles
15. Maple syrup
16. Melons
17. Bananas
18. Butter
19. Salad dressings
20. Milkshakes
21. Cupcakes
22. Nuts
23. Pizza
24. Fried food
25. Microwave popcorn

A7

Low-Carb/Low Glycemic Load Vegetables

Glycemic Index for each food determines the speed sugar is absorbed into the blood. The glycemic index uses a scale from 0 to 100, where 100 is pure glucose. Foods with a high glycemic index, 70 or above, release glucose rapidly and tend to inhibit weight reduction. Low glycemic foods cause a slow, steady digestion, which prevents you from getting hungry. A lower number on the glycemic rating, 55 or below, curtails sugar cravings and helps promote weight reduction. Foods with a rating in the mid-50s to mid-60s are considered average and deemed not to have much impact on blood sugar levels.

It's important to understand how foods affect blood sugar levels. This means knowing both how and how quickly glucose enters the bloodstream. A separate value known as the glycemic load gives a more accurate indication of food's impact on blood sugar. The glycemic load strives to balance the glycemic index with the amount of carbohydrates in each food.

A food's glycemic load is calculated by taking its glycemic index, dividing by one hundred, and multiplying it by the grams of carbohydrates. A glycemic load below 11 is deemed low, a range between

11 through 19 is considered average, and anything above 20 is viewed as high.

Watermelon is atypical because it has a high glycemic index (above 70), yet a low glycemic load of 4.

The list below are vegetables with low carbs and low glycemic loads. They are listed in alphabetical order.

- Artichoke/artichoke hearts
- Asparagus
- Avocado
- Bamboo shoots
- Bean sprouts
- Bell peppers
- Bok choy (sometimes called Chinese cabbage or Pak-choi)
- Broccoli
- Brussels sprouts
- Cabbage (or sauerkraut)
- Cauliflower
- Celery
- Chard
- Cucumber
- Hearty greens: collards, kale, mustard greens, etc.
- Jicama
- Leeks
- Mushrooms
- Nori
- Okra
- Onions
- Peppers (all varieties)
- Radishes
- Scallions or green onions
- Spinach
- Spaghetti squash
- Turnip
- Water chestnuts
- Zucchini

A8

High-Carb/High Glycemic Load Vegetables

The primary vegetables to avoid when reducing carbohydrates are starchier/high sugar veggies listed below.

- Beets
- Carrots
- Corn
- Peas
- Plantains
- Acorn squash

- Butternut squash
- Sweet potato
- Sweet onions
- Eggplant
- Green beans

A9

Low Glycemic Load Fruits

Fruit is an area where many of the low-carb diets differ, as some depend more on the glycemic index or glycemic load, while others just look at total carbs. Also, many diets don't allow any fruits in the first phase of weight reduction. What's the difference between glycemic load and glycemic index? Glycemic load is a ranking method that measures *the amount of carbohydrates* in a serving of food. The glycemic index indicates *how quickly a carbohydrate is broken down* into sugar and released into the blood stream. The list below is not exhaustive and does not take into consideration the carb count.

- Apples
- Apricots
- Blackberries
- Blueberries
- Cantaloupe
- Cherries
- Cranberries (fresh, unsweetened)
- Grapefruit
- Guava

- Lemon
- Limes
- Papaya
- Peach
- Plums
- Raspberries
- Rhubarb
- Strawberries
- Watermelon

A10

High Glycemic Index Fruits

Foods that have a high glycemic index rating of 70 or higher quickly elevate blood sugar. If you are on a weight-reduction program, you'll want to avoid or limit fruits with a high sugar content and glycemic index. These fruits are listed below. Again, it's a partial list and not all inclusive.

- Bananas
- Dates
- Dried fruit
- Figs
- Grapes
- Kiwi
- Lychee

- Mango
- Orange juice
- Persimmons
- Pineapple
- Pomegranate
- Prunes
- Tangerines

Shift Your Mindset to Achieve Better Health

How Can I Start Living a Healthier Lifestyle After Being Unhealthy for So Long?
Transcription of You Tube Video published on September 6, 2017

by Lisa Nichols, Founder and
CEO of Motivating the Masses

You know, so many times we look at health, I know I did, from a topical perspective. And, while it does manifest in our weight gain or weight loss, it manifests in our muscle mass, it manifests in our BMI, it manifests in our body function. I think that's the result of something else.

For me, I'm not a health professional. I'm not a fitness guru. I'm not a nutritionist. I'm a woman who lived really unhealthy for a very long time. And then shifted her mindset and her behaviors and now is walking in a new reality. That's what I am. So, I want to be very clear. And so, the space I came from I think is different than a nutritionist or a fitness expert. But I would love for them to begin to adopt this perspective because you're not working with a half of person that just has weight gain, you're not working with a half of a person that just has a high BMI. You're not working with a quarter of a person that who just has poor eating habits.

If we look at the 360-person and where our behaviors come from—all of your behaviors came from an emotional state of being. An emotional state of being comes from a mindset. So, you think a thing, you feel it, and then you act on it.

And so, we talk about living unhealthy for so long, I love the broadness of it because people think it's just physical, but unhealthy is, oh by the way, my mindset was unconsciously unhealthy. And the unhealthy mindset led to unhealthy habits, led to an unhealthy life-style, led to unhealthy results—hashtag, I was over eighty pounds, I was eighty pounds overweight—because it was a mindset first.

So, I know it's not the fun stuff. We want to jump in and do the crunches. And jump in and do the crash diet. Jump in and do the detox because we want to lose the weight. And I never sling-shotted back up-and-down with my weight. I never even lost it. I wasn't even in a space where I could sling-shot. But, that happens to a number of people. And then some of us hold on to it.

I believe that when you go to what did your weight and what did the unhealthy lifestyle give you? Did it give you an escape? Was it a comfort zone? Was it something that you needed in the moment? And to ask yourself that you have to go to the front of it and what started it. What started it? What started this? Is it my need to serve everyone else? And then, this was the way I served me. Or, was it putting everyone else in front of me and putting myself last? And by the time I got to my needs, I had no energy left.

Was it the need to be loved by everybody? What were those things? What was it for me? It was being significantly hurt in a rela-tionship and putting this jacket on called an eighty-pound weight. I had an eighty-pound jacket on called weight. And it was my com-fort zone.

It allowed me to not have to completely show up. I was ... my body brought me attention that brought me pain. So, then I thought I put this eighty-pound jacket on and then I don't have to worry about that. So, that was my band-aid.

So, what was the thought, the belief, the hurt? What was the fear? What was the anger or the frustration that caused the mindset to lean into emotion, to lean into behavior? I know no one wants to do that. I'd rather get on the treadmill. But I promise you, if you've ever been on a treadmill before and lost weight and then you gained it back or you stopped.

For me, I would stop, start clean. Stop, start clean. I would stop, start clean because the treadmill didn't give me the emotional healing that I was looking for. The carrots and the celery didn't give me the confidence that I had lost when I ended my abusive relationship.

The Weight Watchers, or the Jenny Craig, or the Herbal Life, or the whatever the hell I was doing. There's nothing wrong with those programs. The reason why they didn't work for me is because I wasn't convinced yet that I was worthy of having that result.

So, I know we want it to be something we can touch, and emotions are not something you can touch. And, a mindset is something you can't touch. But I promise you, if you go to the core of your mindset and then the emotion that's sitting right next to it, and we address that, and heal that. Ask yourself the question, "Why did I step into this unhealthy lifestyle? Why did I put on this weight? Why did I go to the refrigerator for comfort? Why did I put so many people in front of me? What was I looking for? What did I need?" With no judgment of yourself. No judgment of yourself. 'Cause you only did what you did based on what you knew.

Now we're seeking to learn more. To know more. We're in a much healthier place than we've ever been. So. Let's ask those questions. For me, the answer was, um, I have two answers: One, I didn't know how to live in the body that I have. It was a body that attracted a lot of attention. And I wasn't sexually mature enough for all the attention that I received in my twenties. And so, it brought me a lot of hurt and pain because I thought every, every room called love was entered through a door called intimacy. And, everyone was promising love, and all, I was having was this form, this version of intimacy, that didn't serve me because it wasn't what I wanted, because it didn't end in a healthy relationship.

And then the other side was I wanted to be accepted when I walked into room by the women in the room. And then, that other body and this personality, there was this gaze, and I wanted the embrace. And so, when I put on this eighty-plus-pound jacket the men stopped coming after me and the women began to befriend me more.

So, I got this false victory that I was looking for. And so, that was my reason, that was my need, was to be liked. And my need was to own my divinity as a woman and the beautiful body, I didn't have that. And so, I had to learn how to own beauty inside and outside. Then, I had to learn how to feel whole and complete when I stepped into a room regardless of the response to me. Those were my emotional needs. That's where I needed to grow. And, when I was able to grow in that area, then I asked myself, based on that, "Are you ready to release the jacket?" And the answer was "Yes."

And then the last thing, I had to kill my ego and ask for help. And really surrender to the fact that I needed help. And so, how do you move into healthier habits? First, give yourself the emotional healing around your weight. Hold on to every part of your body. Hold on to every piece and thank it for its journey that it brought you to. And then, apologize to it. Apologize to it for all the times you band-aided what it needed with what you were able to give it in the moment. Because you just didn't know.

And then, choose this time to change directions, making the last direction okay. But, to change directions and ask in the most humble, open way, ask for help. Not to do the difficult thing, but do the necessary thing, over and over and over again, because I commit to you if you do that necessary thing, over and over and over again, your consistency will get the results that you're looking for.

So, don't ask to start the race fast. Ask someone who can run a marathon with you to walk beside you, whoever that person might be. And then, ask them to hold you to be accountable to the woman or man you choose to become. And then, give yourself permission to get tired, to stop, to get back up, to press reset.

It doesn't matter if it's been five years or twenty-five years. Can you see yourself in an amazing, healthy body and healthy lifestyle, with beauty that takes your own breath away? Because if you can see her, and if you can see him, they've been waiting on you, waiting for you to come home. And when you see that, just walk toward the you you've always known yourself to be. Because this current condition is just the jacket you needed for a period of time. And when the period of time is done, thank it, thank it, and then release it.

About the Author

In July 2016, David Medansky weighed 217 pounds. His doctor told him to lose weight or find another physician, because he didn't want David dying of a heart attack on his watch. Within four months, Medansky dropped 50 pounds and now weighs 167. Being an author, he decided to write about his incredible weight-reduction journey to inspire and help others achieve their weight-reduction goals.

Born and raised in the Chicago metropolitan area, Medansky graduated from the University of Arizona School of Law in 1991. He practiced family law in Phoenix, Arizona until 2004, when he took up the pen to create thriller/suspense novels set in Sin City, otherwise known as Las Vegas.

A bestselling author, Medansky's books are based on his experiences in Las Vegas, his legal background, and his interest in gangsters.

He lives in the Phoenix metropolitan area with his wife.

www.DiscoverYourThinnerSelf.com

"Twenty years from now you will be more disappointed by the things that you didn't do than by the ones you did do."

—Mark Twain

DISCOVER YOUR THINNER SELF

Isn't it time you started your weight-reduction journey today? *Here's to your success for a thinner, healthier you.*

Thanks so much for reading **Discover Your Thinner Self**. One of the most rewarding things about writing is building a relationship with my readers. Your opinion and feedback matters to me, so feel free to reach out and send me an email to **david@dbmedansky.com**. I'd love to know what you think.

I would be honored if you would write an honest review on Amazon, Goodreads, or both. If you liked the book or found it helpful, please consider linking to the review from your social media sites. The best endorsement an author can ask for is enthusiastic, word-of-mouth recommendations from satisfied readers.

With gratitude and to your success,
David Medansky

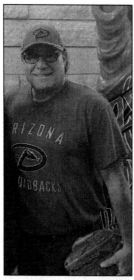 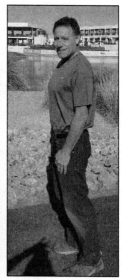

Before at 217 Pounds   After at 162 Pounds
You Too Can Have A Dramatic Transformation!

158

The key to your weight reduction success is your Encore –
It's what you do after you've shed the pounds.

David is available to speak at your event. You can reach the author at:

www.BeyondLosingWeight.com
(602) 721-5218
Email: david@dbmedansky.com

Buy More, Save More

If you're interested in bulk purchases (ten or more copies) of *Discover Your Thinner self*, we offer an aggressive discount schedule. Please call us at (602) 721-5218, or send an email to david@ dbmedansky.com.

For more information contact us at:

www.BeyondLosingWeight.com
(602) 721-5218
Email: david@dbmedansky.com

Acknowledgements

Special thanks to Dr. Frank Agnone who started me on a successful weight-reduction journey after years of failing. And to Cheri Henry, his office manager and HCG administrator who was happy I proved her wrong when it came to me reducing my weight.

I want to acknowledge numerous special people who have influenced my life. They might not remember me, but I remember them as well as the valuable lessons they taught: T. Harv Eker, Blair Singer, Robert Kiyosaki, Kevin Harrington, Jill Lublin, Cheri Tree, Sandra Yancey, Bill Bartmann, and Joel Weldon. I've learned so much from you, and want to acknowledge how much just meeting you and participating in your programs have impacted my life.

In addition, I want to acknowledge and thank Dean Cain (*Superman*), who is a true super human being, for his encouragement during our interview and for the genuine, kind and generous person I know him to be. Dean, thank you. Your support, sincerity and willingness to help others is greatly appreciated.

To Mike Koenigs whose presentation at Author 101 University gave me the inspiration to write this book.

To Craig Duswalt who encouraged me to go beyond losing weight and do so much more to help others with weight issues.

To John Fontana for providing stories and material to assist me in communicating my message.

To David Chilton, author of *The Wealthy Barber*, for creating and sharing "The Chilton Method" to market, promote, and sell books. The Chilton Method taught me just how much I didn't know about marketing this book.

To Rachel Smartt for introducing me to Juice Plus and all its wonderful health benefits. And for her encouragement and support throughout this endeavor.

To Leeza Gibbons, your words of advice, "Warmth is the currency of influence," and "A little pivot can give you different optics," resonated with me and improved my life. Thank you.

To Jeff Hoffman, Co-founder, Priceline.com, thank you for inspiring me to take ten minutes each day and challenge myself to learn one new thing that I don't necessarily need to know.

Information about Jenny Craig printed with the company's written permission and authorization.

Enroll Now!

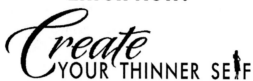

CREATE YOUR THINNER SELF WEIGHT REDUCTION ONLINE COURSE

A self-guided, practical, and common-sense approach to weight loss that holds you accountable.

Lose Weight in 30 days or less by improving your eating habits and lifestyle.

Outcome: By the end of the program you will:

- Create body weight reduction goals and start to see a downshift in your weight.
- Develop healthier eating habits. Improve from making unhealthy food choices to healthier, budget friendly, nutritious, and great tasting choices that won't take a lot of time to prepare.
- Connect with a support group to keep you accountable.
- You may consider reviewing your wardrobe, and update it with some new choices, reflecting how good you feel with your weight loss, or get a makeover.
- You'll feel better, you'll have more energy, and may even sleep better.

- Your overall health might improve (Medical advice, however, is NOT given and you should consult your doctor before starting any weight loss program).

When you take the course, do the work, and don't get the results you want, David Medansky will get on the phone with you for one-on-one coaching or live support to make sure you get results.

If you're ready to invest in yourself and take advantage of this exclusive opportunity, go to www.BeyondLosingWeight.com for more information.

Limited seating. Additional fees and tuition may apply at the time of registration. This offer can be withdrawn earlier if the program sells out or is no longer being offered. David Medansky and Beyond Losing Weight LLC reserves the right to refuse admission, and to remove from the program anyone it believes is disrupting the course.

CPSIA information can be obtained
at www.ICGtesting.com
Printed in the USA
FFOW01n0015201217
44175212-43577FF